THE
EVERYTHING.
GUIDE TO
HASHIMOTO'S
THYROIDITIS

Dear Reader,

After struggling for more than a decade with Hashimoto's thyroiditis, and spending much of that floundering without a clear path to wellness, I couldn't be more passionate about helping people avoid the same frustration. What felt like an impossible climb out of fatigue, endless weight gain, and depression actually became a stunning transformation. Within 6 months of utilizing the protocols outlined in this book, I had lost more than 50 pounds and felt like a brand-new person. Within a year I had gone from a size 16 to a size 2, became a runner, and started doing yoga. This dramatic change is what inspired me to become a nutritionist.

I've found that as long as I maintain my lifestyle of body-focused wellness and my thyroid-friendly Paleo diet, I do not have relapses back into the debilitating fatigue and depression that ruled my life for so long. While it's been years since I experienced the crushing weight of uncontrolled Hashimoto's, I will never forget how it felt to be so helpless when it came to understanding my body. I hope that this book will help you fast-track your way to a place of health, healing, and renewed vitality!

Aimee McNew, MNT

Welcome to the EVERYTHING® Series!

These handy, accessible books give you all you need to tackle a difficult project, gain a new hobby, comprehend a fascinating topic, prepare for an exam, or even brush up on something you learned back in school but have since forgotten.

You can choose to read an Everything® book from cover to cover or just pick out the information you want from our four useful boxes: e-questions, e-facts, e-alerts, and e-ssentials.

We give you everything you need to know on the subject, but throw in a lot of fun stuff along the way, too.

We now have more than 400 Everything® books in print, spanning such wide-ranging categories as weddings, pregnancy, cooking, music instruction, foreign language, crafts, pets, New Age, and so much more. When you're done reading them all, you can finally say you know Everything®!

QUESTION

Answers to common questions

FACT

Important snippets of information

ALERT

Urgent warnings

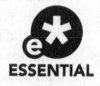

ESSENTIAL

Quick handy tips

PUBLISHER Karen Cooper

MANAGING EDITOR Lisa Laing

COPY CHIEF Casey Ebert

ASSISTANT PRODUCTION EDITOR Jo-Anne Duhamel

ACQUISITIONS EDITOR Hillary Thompson

DEVELOPMENT EDITOR Hillary Thompson

EVERYTHING® SERIES COVER DESIGNER Erin Alexander

Visit the entire Everything® series at www.everything.com

THE EVERYTHING®

GUIDE TO HASHIMOTO'S THYROIDITIS

A healing plan for managing symptoms naturally

Aimee McNew, MNT

Adams Media
New York London Toronto Sydney New Delhi

In loving memory of my grandmother,
RoseMarie Brunton (1942–2012), whose constant voice of encouragement
for both my writing and my quest for wellness helped to make me who I am.

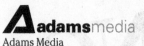

Adams Media
An Imprint of Simon & Schuster, Inc.
100 Technology Center Drive
Stoughton, MA 02072

An Everything® Series Book.
Everything® and everything.com® are registered trademarks of Simon & Schuster, Inc.

ADAMS MEDIA and colophon are trademarks of Simon and Schuster.

For information about special discounts for bulk purchases, please contact Simon & Schuster Special Sales at 1-866-506-1949 or business@simonandschuster.com.

The Simon & Schuster Speakers Bureau can bring authors to your live event. For more information or to book an event contact the Simon & Schuster Speakers Bureau at 1-866-248-3049 or visit our website at www.simonspeakers.com.

Nutritional statistics by Melinda Boyd, MPH, MHR, RD.
Manufactured in the United States of America

7 2022

Library of Congress Cataloging-in-Publication Data has been applied for.

ISBN 978-1-4405-9814-2
ISBN 978-1-4405-9815-9 (ebook)

This book is intended as general information only, and should not be used to diagnose or treat any health condition. In light of the complex, individual, and specific nature of health problems, this book is not intended to replace professional medical advice. The ideas, procedures, and suggestions in this book are intended to supplement, not replace, the advice of a trained medical professional. Consult your physician before adopting any of the suggestions in this book, as well as about any condition that may require diagnosis or medical attention. The author and publisher disclaim any liability arising directly or indirectly from the use of this book.

Always follow safety and commonsense cooking protocol while using kitchen utensils, operating ovens and stoves, and handling uncooked food. If children are assisting in the preparation of any recipe, they should always be supervised by an adult.

Contains material adapted from *The Everything® Paleolithic Diet Book* by Jodie Cohen and Gilaad Cohen, copyright © 2011 by Simon & Schuster, Inc., ISBN 978-1-4405-1206-3; *The Everything® Weeknight Paleo Cookbook* by Michelle Fagone, copyright © 2014 by Simon & Schuster, Inc., ISBN 978-1-4405-7229-6; and *The Everything® Vegan Paleo Cookbook* by Daelyn Fortney, copyright © 2015 by Simon & Schuster, Inc., ISBN 978-1-4405-9022-1.

Contents

Acknowledgments

Writing a book with a newborn seems like the silliest thing in the world, but I want to thank my husband, Marvin, who believes in me more than I often believe in myself, and my son, Harry, who made his mama smile through the sleepless nights and brainless days of caring for an infant while writing a book. I would also like to thank my mom and my friend Molly for always being willing to hold the baby so I could write. Thanks also to Travis Thrasher, for his invaluable insight and advice.

Special thanks to Hillary and the awesome team at F+W Media and Adams Media for the opportunity to write on a topic that I'm so passionate about.

Introduction

HASHIMOTO'S THYROIDITIS AFFECTS MORE than 14 million Americans, and a majority of those are women. Thus, autoimmune thyroid disease has become a widespread issue in women's health. Conventional medical treatments have proven largely ineffective, especially where quality of life is concerned. Thyroid levels may look normal on paper, but patients with Hashimoto's know that there is more to this disease than meets the eye.

There is much speculation as to why autoimmune diseases of all kinds are on the rise, but the latest research all seems to point toward gut health and the microbiome—the bacterial landscape of our intestines that strongly impacts digestion and the immune system. Autoimmune disorders happen when the immune system goes awry. Recovery begins not just when we offer hormone replacement, but when we address the root cause of the issue. For Hashimoto's, this often requires a multifaceted approach with dietary and lifestyle changes, as well as hormone replacement.

With the rise of the Paleo diet, many are seeing health benefits that far surpass weight loss alone, including restoration and remission from autoimmune disorders such as Hashimoto's. While critics of the Paleo diet abound, research is proving that it is therapeutic for chronic conditions because it reduces systemic inflammation, balances cholesterol, aids in weight loss, and eliminates autoimmune-triggering foods such as gluten, soy, and dairy.

Paleo, of course, goes far beyond the basics of a simple "use it and lose it" dietary approach. It's a lifestyle change best implemented as a long-term dietary protocol. Principles of the Paleo diet go far and above the overly simplified "eat like a caveman" mantra that critics insist is hard to follow. The Paleo diet is about clean eating and clean living. It encourages a toxin-free home, as well as an organic, whole-food diet that is easy on the digestive system. Contrary to popular belief, whole grains are actually quite hard to digest, and frankly, vegetables are a richer source of fiber and nutrients than whole wheat ever could be.

Hashimoto's thyroiditis is a disease that can easily ruin the quality of a person's life, but by taking a holistic, integrated approach, sufferers can experience relief and a return to the normalcy of pre-Hashimoto's days. This book places in your hands a complete path to healing, including ways to advocate for yourself as a patient, which is essential. With your unique set of conditions and health history, learning to talk the talk and listen to what your body is saying become valuable assets when communicating with your healthcare providers and in assessing which protocols and foods are helpful and which are not.

While there is no easy way to go about making the major lifestyle changes that are involved with transitioning to a Paleo diet and toxin-free living, the good news is that healing is a journey that is not meant to happen overnight. There is no race to the finish line when it comes to working your way toward wellness, and, in fact, approaching the process with set time frames in mind typically leads to frustration and setbacks. If you acknowledge that your body's autoimmune breakdown didn't happen instantly, and that the body often takes as long (or longer) to heal as it did to get sick, then you will be able to give yourself the freedom to adjust to this new way of living without the burden of impossible expectations. That being said, while healing doesn't happen immediately, you will notice plenty of positive effects in the early days of Paleo living that will bolster your desire to keep moving forward—things like better sleep, clothes that fit better, and improved energy levels, to name a few. Those are things to get excited about, and celebrating each small victory as it comes will make this lifestyle change feel both effortless and effective.

CHAPTER 1

What Is Hashimoto's Thyroiditis?

Autoimmune thyroid disease, including Hashimoto's thyroiditis, is the most common autoimmune disorder that exists, according to *Endocrine Reviews*. It now affects a whopping 14 million people in the United States alone, or about 4 percent of the total population. The *Journal of Immunology Research* notes that of all autoimmune cases, 30 percent are of thyroid autoimmunity. Because it impacts such a small slice of the American population, Hashimoto's is classed as a rare disease, but unfortunately, it is often misdiagnosed or goes undiagnosed for years.

The Butterfly Organ

The thyroid is an endocrine gland, which means that it produces hormones. It is located in the lower part of the neck and sits a little lower than the Adam's apple, and measures about 2" in length. It is shaped like an H, but is also referred to as the butterfly organ because of its similarity in shape.

While the thyroid is a relatively small organ, it regulates a huge percentage of body function because it controls metabolism, or the body's energy supply. When the thyroid isn't working as it should, it affects several body systems and symptoms are widespread.

The thyroid makes two different hormones: thyroxine, or T4, and triiodothyronine, or T3. T4 is an inactive form of T3, and T3 is produced when body cells activate the T4. The body's thyroid hormone production is spurred by the efforts of another endocrine gland, the pituitary, which is located in the brain. The pituitary produces TSH, or thyroid-stimulating hormone, and that instructs the thyroid to produce more T4. The communication between endocrine glands is meant to be effortless, but sadly, hormones are susceptible to many interruptions, and even slight imbalances with other body systems can cause chaos as well as over- or underproduction of hormones. The thyroid is especially sensitive.

Underproduction of thyroid hormone is referred to as hypothyroidism, and overproduction as hyperthyroidism. Both can be a result of several factors that are not autoimmune in nature, but the most common kind of thyroid disorder is Hashimoto's, or autoimmune hypothyroid disease.

The Immune System and Autoimmune Disease

The immune system is thought to be the protective body force that keeps germs away, or at least eradicates them when they do enter the body. About 70 percent of the immune system resides in the gut in the form of gut-associated lymphoid tissue (GALT). Autoimmune disease is triggered when the gut becomes imbalanced or overwhelmed with toxins, pathogens, or bacteria that break down the barrier function of the intestines. As a result of this weakened barrier, particles not intended to enter the bloodstream make their way throughout the body. The presence of these particles does not go unnoticed, and it is the immune system that sounds the alarm. However, instead of being able to recognize that the particles are foreign, the immune system makes associations with the closest thing that it recognizes so that it can produce antibodies to combat the "disease." Unfortunately, in cases of autoimmunity, this results in the immune system mounting an attack against its own body. There are more than eighty varieties of autoimmune diseases, according to the research of Johns Hopkins Medicine. Thyroid diseases make up just two of those eighty.

FACT

A goiter is swelling of the thyroid gland as a result of inflammation or iodine deficiency. In the United States, goiters are most often a result of autoimmune thyroid disease. Goiters can be reduced in many cases by managing autoimmunity, as well as by proper thyroid hormone replacement. In some more extreme cases, goiters may need to be surgically removed.

The immune system becomes weaponized in cases of autoimmune disease because it finds similarities between the foreign particles that have entered the bloodstream and specific organs or tissues that are present in the body. Some of this is determined by genetic susceptibility, but some of it is also determined by the specific particles that are in the blood. Dairy and gluten, for example, closely resemble thyroid tissue when they are broken down to the cellular level. When the immune system "finds" these particles in the bloodstream, it gets the message that the thyroid is trying to take over the whole body. Being the body's line of defense, the immune system is activated and launches an antibody attack against the thyroid to put it back in its place. As a result, thyroid function is suppressed. If dietary changes are not made, the immune system continues to attack the thyroid, in some cases resulting in total destruction of the gland's ability to produce hormones. Continued autoimmune activation against the thyroid can also result in high levels of inflammation that can result in a goiter, which is enlargement of the thyroid gland.

The Basics of Thyroid Disease

There are three varieties of thyroid disease: Graves' disease, postpartum thyroiditis, and Hashimoto's thyroiditis. Postpartum thyroiditis does become Hashimoto's in about 20 percent of cases.

While these factors may not be present in all cases of thyroid disease (i.e., not everyone who has autoimmune thyroid disease will be diagnosed with a visible goiter), some or all of these are commonly found in all three types of thyroid disease:

- An overactive immune system
- Swelling in the gland (goiter)
- Genetic predisposition
- Requires medical treatment in some capacity (does not go away on its own)
- Changes in menstrual cycles for women
- Mood changes such as anxiety or depression
- Changes in libido

There are, however, some distinct differences among these three types of autoimmune thyroid activation:

- Graves' and Hashimoto's are often diagnosed between the ages of 40 and 60, while postpartum thyroiditis generally occurs within 12 months after pregnancy.
- Graves' results in weight loss and increased body heat, while Hashimoto's and postpartum have the opposite effect—weight gain (usually 10–20 pounds) or the inability to lose weight, as well as sensitivity to cold or chilly extremities.
- Graves' disease causes an overproduction of thyroid hormone by the body and is often treated with radiated iodine, beta blockers, or antithyroid medications. In some cases, part or all of the thyroid must be removed. Hashimoto's and postpartum require additional thyroid hormone, and are treated with thyroid hormone replacement and additional nutrient supplementation.

Hashimoto's Thyroiditis

Hashimoto's thyroiditis is the most common form of thyroid disease, affecting women 7–10 times more than men. Of those who develop the disease, an immune defect is present in most, along with a genetic predisposition that is triggered by environmental or hormonal factors (or both).

Hashimoto's often develops slowly over time, with symptoms presenting so gradually as to almost be imperceptible at first. Over time, perhaps even years, symptoms can become irritating or unmanageable. Unfortunately, Hashimoto's is frequently misdiagnosed or undiagnosed, leaving patients suffering for months or years until their symptoms become so pronounced that doctors take a second or third look.

Hashimoto's thyroiditis and nonautoimmune hypothyroidism can often be confused. Doctors will often run only one or two of the entire panel of tests needed to properly diagnose autoimmunity, and thus will diagnose hypothyroidism and prescribe thyroid hormone replacement. In some cases, this can be enough to address the disease for a while, since hormone replacement is a key part of addressing Hashimoto's. But in many cases, hormone replacement alone is insufficient, resulting in symptoms that do not go away and a disease that continues to worsen.

Causes, Triggers, and Risk Factors of Hashimoto's Thyroiditis

Hashimoto's, like any other autoimmune disease, is complex and multifaceted and is still the subject of research. Medical science doesn't quite have definitive answers on every aspect of the disease, but what is known is that there are several associated causes, triggers, and risk factors.

CAUSES
- Having a current autoimmune disease, particularly if it is uncontrolled
- Pregnancy
- Genetic predisposition (HLA-DR3 or HLA-DR5)

TRIGGERS
- Excessive iodine intake
- Chemical or pesticide exposure and similar environmental factors
- Viral infections
- Bacterial infections
- Treatment with certain medications
- Hormonal fluctuation such as in puberty, pregnancy, or menopause

- Having another autoimmune disorder, especially rheumatoid arthritis or type 1 diabetes
- Being a woman
- Being in the 30–50 age range
- Having a parent, sibling, aunt, uncle, or grandparent with Hashimoto's or any autoimmune disease

ALERT

Most people with Hashimoto's only have a small slice of triggers, causes, or risk factors. Even just one is enough for Hashimoto's to be present, and rarely will people have all the possible factors. If you suspect that you have Hashimoto's, speak to your doctor about being tested, and don't give up if the results are not conclusive initially. Hashimoto's is frequently misdiagnosed.

Signs and Symptoms of Hashimoto's Thyroiditis

Hashimoto's has a wide range of symptoms that can present at any stage of the disease, and unfortunately most are not diagnosed until a number of these are present. That being said, some patients can have Hashimoto's without symptoms of hypothyroidism, or only one or two symptoms from this list:

- Fatigue
- Weight gain
- Inability to lose weight
- Constipation
- Sensitivity to cold
- Dry skin
- Depression
- Muscle aches or cramps
- Joint pain
- Reduced activity tolerance
- Irregular or extremely heavy periods

- Goiter
- Difficulty swallowing not associated with sore throat
- Reduced concentration or mental acuity
- Dry or brittle nails
- Dry or brittle hair
- Hair loss
- Inability to conceive
- Recurrent early miscarriage
- Decreased basal body temperature
- Decreased average heart rate
- Decreased blood pressure
- Elevated LDL cholesterol
- Drowsiness
- Lack of restorative sleep
- Insomnia
- Mood swings
- Anxiety
- Hoarseness
- Difficulty breathing
- Tenderness or pain in the thyroid area or lower neck
- Chest pain
- Increased susceptibility to colds or other infections

ESSENTIAL

Having trouble getting a doctor to run the correct labs for assessing thyroid health? You live in the golden age of health information, and several patient-ordered lab companies exist so that you can have a say in your own medical information. On these sites you can order your own labs, retrieve results, and even find basic interpretation. Two of the most popular patient-driven lab companies, LabCorp and Quest Diagnostics, have locations all across the United States and offer reasonably priced tests. A word of caution: if you are ordering your own labs, insurance often won't cover it, so be sure to check with them first.

Getting Diagnosed

If you visit your doctor and have a number of symptoms associated with Hashimoto's or hypothyroidism, chances are you will be tested for TSH, or thyroid-stimulating hormone. This hormone can be useful as part of a diagnosis for Hashimoto's, but a proper diagnosis and assessment of the state of the thyroid requires other labs. According to the *Textbook of Natural Medicine*, which promotes a more integrative, preventive approach to disease, effective screening for and diagnosis of Hashimoto's should include thyroid regulation marker (the aforementioned TSH), along with thyroid output (free T3 and free T4), as well as thyroid inflammatory markers (antibodies). The following labs should be used to diagnose Hashimoto's or to monitor disease progression and remission:

- **Free T3: T3, or triiodothyronine,** is the active form of the thyroid hormone that circulates in the blood bound to proteins that transport it through the body. The free T3 measurement analyzes the portion of T3 that is not connected to carrier proteins, and thus is available for biological action, or is bioavailable. Measuring T3 can have highly variable results, as the number of proteins available for transport will vary. Free T3, however, is a more consistent result because the levels available for biological action are kept as consistent as possible within the body. When Hashimoto's is present, this is not the case, and thus measuring free T3 can help to assess disease management.

- **Free T4: T4, also known as thyroxine,** is the inactive thyroid hormone that gets converted to active form when needed. Free T4 is a blood test that measures the bioavailable T4, or the portion of T4 that is freely accessible by tissues for conversion into T3. Most practitioners consider free T4 to be the primary lab test for assessing true thyroid function, but only in the context of other lab results, like free T3 and TSH.

- **TSH: TSH, or thyroid-stimulating hormone,** is a hormone produced by the pituitary gland to stimulate the thyroid to make more hormones. In undiagnosed Hashimoto's, TSH is elevated due to the pituitary gland's attempts to force the thyroid to hear its message. In Hashimoto's patients who are being treated with hormone replacement, TSH will register on the low end of normal, or even significantly lower, since the pituitary doesn't need to tell the thyroid to produce more hormones, if any at all.

- **Thyroglobulin antibody:** A blood test that checks for the presence of a specific antibody that attacks the thyroid, this test is one of two used to confirm the presence of an immune reaction and therefore a confirmation of Hashimoto's thyroiditis. As Hashimoto's is treated with thyroid replacement hormone and lifestyle adjustments, these antibody levels will decrease and potentially reach the normal range.

- **Thyroid peroxidase antibody:** Another blood test that checks for the presence of antibodies that are attacking the thyroid. When one or both thyroid antibodies that were out of range and used to diagnose Hashimoto's return to normal levels, it is said that the person is in remission. Because autoimmune disease never goes away, a person can develop increased antibodies again, usually due to outside factors, changes in thyroid medication, or hormonal changes.

- **Reverse T3:** This is literally the opposite of T3. While free T3 is the bioavailable form of T3, reverse T3 is T4 that instead of being converted to active hormone is stored away as reverse T3. This can happen when the body is under stress and cells attempt to conserve energy by converting less T4 to T3. Reverse T3 can also be a result of low iron levels, which are required for optimal thyroid hormone activation. Whereas free T3 is responsible for normalizing metabolic function, especially in those who have Hashimoto's and are taking a T4 and T3 hormone replacement, reverse T3 actually decreases metabolic function and can produce symptoms of hypothyroidism even if free T3 and free T4 levels look optimal. While this one isn't essential for diagnosis, it is helpful in monitoring treatment progress of Hashimoto's, including effectiveness of hormone replacement and other aggravating factors.

Additionally, thyroid ultrasound can be used to assess damage done to thyroid tissue, but this is less common unless there are other complications associated with the disease.

Unfortunately, as things currently are, thyroid screening is not routine beyond checking TSH for anyone who presents with possible hypothyroid symptoms, especially women in their thirties and forties. Because of this, many cases of Hashimoto's can go undiagnosed for years or even decades. Those who have other autoimmune conditions or hormone irregularities will likely receive a faster diagnosis for Hashimoto's because of more in-depth testing. Unfortunately, this is still not preventive and most who are diagnosed with Hashimoto's may suffer for years with treatable symptoms or avoidable complications. One example is recurrent pregnancy loss due to Hashimoto's thyroiditis. It is not common to screen pregnant women for Hashimoto's, and as such, a woman experiencing miscarriage or inability to conceive will usually not be tested until it has been problematic for quite some time. In the United States it is common for OB-GYNs to not investigate causes of miscarriage until three consecutive pregnancy losses have happened.

ESSENTIAL

If you've newly been diagnosed with Hashimoto's or have recently begun taking thyroid hormone replacement medication, it's important to have regular and frequent thyroid lab testing done. The thyroid can be volatile, and especially in the presence of autoimmune reactions, a great deal of yo-yoing may take place in the first weeks and months. Monitoring thyroid labs every 6–8 weeks can provide a less rocky path toward wellness and remission.

The process of getting diagnosed with Hashimoto's can feel long and intense, but you can be proactive by learning to interpret your own labs. Standard lab ranges that are considered normal for thyroid tests are as follows:

- **T4:** 4.8–13.2 mg/dL
- **Free T4:** 0.9–2.0 ng/dL
- **T3:** 80–220 ng/dL
- **Free T3:** 1.4–4.2 pg/mL
- **TSH:** 0.35–5.50 mIU/mL

Keep in mind that practitioners who are proactive in addressing Hashimoto's will work with narrower lab ranges, and even if you fall within these "normal" levels, your thyroid may not be functioning optimally.

What to Do after the Diagnosis

So you're told your body is producing antibodies against your thyroid, and so much starts to become clearer. Symptoms you've had for weeks, months, or even years begin to make sense, and you finally see a path toward relief. Unfortunately, for many, this isn't the case.

Receiving a diagnosis of Hashimoto's thyroiditis is just the first step in a journey toward wellness and remission. Once your body has started to attack itself, there is no simple, overnight fix. A path to healing must be prepared, and for many, this needs to be fluid. The body is complex, and where hormones are concerned, there are too many variables to get it right the first or second time.

QUESTION

What is the first thing I should do after finding out I have Hashimoto's?
Don't panic. That seems simple enough, but honestly: take a deep breath. Finding out that you have autoimmune disease can feel overwhelming. It can feel limiting. It can feel like a prison. Accept the reality, but then move quickly into the belief that you will not be stuck in your diagnosis. Of all autoimmune disorders, Hashimoto's responds very well to hormone and lifestyle treatment. As you learn to listen to your body, your process of healing will become second nature.

After being diagnosed with Hashimoto's, depending on your lab levels, you will likely be prescribed hormone replacement of some kind. Even though you're not a doctor, you do have some say in the medication that you take, so do your research. Consider other lifestyle factors that can be aggravating your autoimmune condition, such as diet and other allergy sources, as well as other factors that can be problematic (think: stress). While recovery from an autoimmune disorder does require some time and effort, it doesn't have to take over your life. Transitioning to a lifestyle of healing for Hashimoto's can happen seamlessly, but it most likely won't happen immediately.

Making Sure You Get the Right Diagnosis

Endocrine disorders are rarely cut and dried, and Hashimoto's is no exception. Receiving a diagnosis can be the first step toward recovery, but an incorrect or partial diagnosis can actually cause more setbacks. It's important to take on the mindset of an explorer who is out to solve the mystery of your body. While you may never receive all the answers, if you become curious, you will be more apt to notice tiny details that can be incredibly helpful to your doctor as you navigate the process of working toward healing.

Questions to explore if you've been diagnosed with Hashimoto's include:

- How far has it progressed regarding permanent damage to my thyroid?
- What aggravating factors are there in my lifestyle, diet, or existing medications that I need to address?
- What positive, health-supporting things am I already incorporating into my lifestyle? What dietary, physical, and mental actions can I add?
- Are there other conditions that I might possibly have that have not yet been diagnosed or explored? Are there other conditions that I am at risk for?
- Are there other tests that should be run or conditions to be monitored to help assess the process of healing?
- How do I know if the thyroid hormone replacement is working?
- How often do my thyroid levels need to be monitored?
- What medications can interfere with thyroid hormone and/or falsely increase or decrease thyroid hormone levels?
- What symptoms are most problematic, and what would indicate a problem or worsening condition?
- How quickly will I be able to lose weight?
- What foods should I avoid as I work toward healing Hashimoto's and the associated condition of increased intestinal permeability (leaky gut)?
- Do I need to do anything to help reduce my level of antibodies, or will they reduce on their own as a result of addressing other factors?
- Are my children at risk of developing this condition?

When it comes to Hashimoto's, you will find that there are primarily two common approaches: conventional and holistic. The mindset of the practitioner who diagnoses you can have a huge impact on the next steps. It is important to ask your doctor how she intends to treat your condition.

In recent years, it has become increasingly popular for practitioners to take an integrative approach to Hashimoto's and autoimmunity in general. This refers to a blended mode of treatment that utilizes both conventional and holistic methods to create a customized path to healing. However, even the best practitioner will never have the personal knowledge that you have of yourself, and that's why becoming involved in the process, and getting to know your diagnosis as well as the factors that make your situation unique from anyone else, will have an immense impact on your path toward healing from Hashimoto's.

CHAPTER 2

The Physical Impact
of Hashimoto's

Autoimmune thyroid disease causes systemic symptoms that can range from mildly irritating to debilitating. Beyond the actual effect that antibodies have on the thyroid gland itself, Hashimoto's can also cause other organs and body systems to malfunction, resulting in a cascade effect of numerous, layered conditions that can make one or all of them difficult to diagnose. With a proper Hashimoto's diagnosis, one layer can be peeled away and other presenting conditions explored. In many cases it can be unclear whether Hashimoto's was the disease that triggered other disorders, or whether it was a result of other conditions or inflammation within the body.

Conditions Related to Hashimoto's

The list of related diseases, disorders, and complications associated with Hashimoto's is quite extensive, but not exhaustive. More research is being done to understand the genetic component in this and many other autoimmune disorders, but for now, any of the following can be present before, during, or after Hashimoto's, with associations that are in some cases not fully understood. Having Hashimoto's is not a guarantee that any of the following will present, nor are any of the following automatic indicators of autoimmune thyroid disease. Bioindividuality plays a strong role in determining who gets each condition and how they are specifically linked within the body. The most commonly associated conditions will be discussed in further detail in this chapter.

- Addison's disease
- Celiac disease
- Cardiovascular disease
- Autoimmune hepatitis
- Infertility
- Rheumatoid arthritis
- Recurrent pregnancy loss
- Type 1 diabetes
- Type 2 diabetes
- Multiple sclerosis
- Lupus
- Sjögren's syndrome
- Pernicious anemia
- Premature ovarian failure
- Thrombocytic purpura
- Vitiligo
- Elevated LDL cholesterol
- Myxedema
- Thyroid lymphoma
- Pregnancy complications
- Fibromyalgia
- Chronic viral infections
- IBS or IBD

- Depression and/or mania
- Sleep disorders and insomnia
- Chronic fatigue syndrome
- Obesity
- Estrogen dominance
- Anxiety disorders and panic attacks

Genetic predisposition plays a large determining role in who gets what autoimmune diseases and other chronic conditions. Evaluating the personal health of your parents, siblings, and grandparents can be a good starting place for living a preventive lifestyle. However, the world in which we live is increasingly more polluted and toxic, and thus, some disease-triggering environmental factors that exist today may not have been present even one or two decades ago. Even if no family history exists, it is still possible to have a genetic component to autoimmune or chronic disease.

The Burden of an Overactive Immune System

When you hear mention of an overactive immune system, you might think that's a good thing. After all, the immune system is what fights off viruses, bacteria, and other invaders, so if the immune system works extra hard that should be good, right? Unfortunately, an overactive immune system, as in the case of autoimmune disease, actually translates into low-functioning immunity. Your immune system is so occupied with producing antibodies against your own organs that it ignores other invaders from the outside, such as viral infections. People with autoimmune or chronic disorders have reduced immunity and are more susceptible to frequent colds, influenza, or other viral and bacterial infections because their immune system is malfunctioning. It is a true case of the body letting its guard down.

Unfortunately, people who have Hashimoto's and other related conditions will often become further rundown due to the body's inability to fend off germs from the outside world, making it even harder for the body to recover from its own internal attack. Additionally, once the immune system is primed to create antibodies for its own organs, it rarely stops at one. Autoimmune disorders tend to stack because of how closely related and communicative the organs are, particularly those of the endocrine system. System-wide disorders such as rheumatoid arthritis, fibromyalgia, lupus, and in the most extreme cases, multiple sclerosis, can set in as a result. Hashimoto's can also come after or at the same time as any of these or multiple other disorders.

Seeking a Gradual Remission

The process of working toward remission from an autoimmune disease is much more complex than suppressing the immune system. Even though the immune system needs to down-regulate its attacks on organs, it needs to become more sensitized to the toxins it's actually intended to fight. This doesn't happen with the flip of a switch, nor is it a straightforward process. Healing from autoimmune disease often comes in the form of one step forward, two steps back, but it's this gradual movement that allows the immune system to reprogram itself over time and for the body's tissue to heal, inflammation to cool, and the protective barriers in the gut wall to once again resume their proper function.

The Adrenal Connection and Chronic Fatigue Syndrome

The adrenal glands sit just above the kidneys and are endocrine organs that produce a variety of hormones. They're about 3" long, and just over 1" wide. The adrenals are divided into two parts—the outer cortex and the inner medulla—both of which produce hormones that have a broad array of effects on the body.

The adrenal cortex produces hormones that are essential for body function, including:

- **Cortisol:** A hormone responsible for your body's stress response as well as how protein, fat, and carbohydrates are converted into usable energy
- **Corticosterone:** A hormone that works with cortisol to manage immune and inflammatory actions and responses within the body

- **Aldosterone:** A hormone that regulates blood pressure as well as electrolyte balance
- **Sex hormones:** Reproductive male and female hormones, such as testosterone and estrogen, are produced in lesser amounts by the adrenal glands, but they are primarily produced in either the testes or ovaries

The inner medulla produces hormones that are less critical for total body function, but they can still have a dramatic impact, as they are aimed at helping your body deal with stress in any of its forms. The adrenal medulla produces hormones that are involved in the infamous fight-or-flight response:

- **Epinephrine:** A hormone more popularly known as adrenaline that floods the body with the tools it needs to immediately respond to sources of stress (e.g., by pulling blood sugar from its stored locations and releasing it into the bloodstream, as well as by elevating heart rate and shuffling extra blood to the brain and the muscles for immediate action)
- **Norepinephrine:** A hormone that works closely with epinephrine in perpetuating the stress response by narrowing blood vessels and increasing blood pressure

Because the adrenals are endocrine organs, they can be extremely susceptible to hormone imbalances elsewhere in the body, particularly with the thyroid. When the thyroid is not functioning optimally, the adrenals often compensate by producing more stress hormones. This cycle results in the adrenals becoming overtaxed, and eventually, they run out of steam. While the thyroid regulates metabolism, the adrenals play a key role in energy production, so when both are outside of their normal and optimal range, the entire body will notice effects, primarily in energy levels.

ESSENTIAL

Adrenal function can be tested via blood or saliva. Saliva produces more accurate results of the hormones that are actually available for your body to use, whereas blood tests reflect how much hormone is circulating, even if it is not bioavailable. You can obtain saliva test kits from your doctor, or you can order them online. Additionally, alternative practitioners such as nutritionists and chiropractors may be able to order these sorts of tests.

Chronic Fatigue Syndrome

Even just a decade ago, chronic fatigue syndrome, or CFS, was thought to be a made-up condition. It was a name given to people who were excessively tired, and had many symptoms associated with other chronic disorders, but which couldn't seem to match up to anything specific. So CFS became the blanket diagnosis for "you're clearly not normal but we don't know what's wrong with you." On the flip side, CFS was rejected by many medical professionals as a quack diagnosis, and even if adrenal fatigue seemed to be present in patients, they would resist offering this possibility, instead leaving their patients without any direction at all.

Many symptoms of CFS match up with symptoms of Hashimoto's. In cases where one condition is addressed, and symptoms continue to present, it is often necessary to support the other. The adrenal glands and the thyroid are three peas in a pod, and it is impossible to ignore one without considering the impact on the other. Consider this list of symptoms for CFS or adrenal fatigue:

- Lack of restful sleep
- Lethargy
- Salt cravings
- Low energy reserves
- Reduced tolerance of stressful situations
- Decreased libido
- Reduced immunity/frequent illness
- Low blood pressure or low blood sugar
- Depression
- Hormonal imbalance
- Lack of clear thinking
- Poor memory
- Sleep disorders and insomnia

Of those symptoms, many overlap with Hashimoto's and other autoimmune conditions, so if Hashimoto's doesn't seem to improve, it is essential to consider the impact that the adrenal glands may be having on total body energy levels and overall wellness.

Weight and Metabolism

One of the most common symptoms of Hashimoto's is weight gain or the inability to lose weight. This is perhaps what most often drives doctors to take a closer look at the thyroid. Unfortunately, what usually happens is that TSH levels are all that is checked. For numerous Hashimoto's patients, these levels can return as "normal," and they are sent away frustrated that their mysterious weight issue has not been solved.

ALERT

Judging a thyroid condition simply by the weight on the scale is a mistake that too many patients make. Hormone replacement may make it easier to lose weight, but in many cases, if lifestyle factors aren't properly adjusted to address autoimmunity, antibodies can actually increase during this time. It is important to prioritize total body health over one slice of it—numbers on the scale aren't truly reflective of internal health when viewed on their own.

Looking into the full panel of thyroid labs often gives more of a clue as to why the scale isn't budging, and it's no wonder, since the thyroid regulates metabolism. With a sluggish or virtually nonexistent metabolism, the body's fuel-burning engines are slowed and weight begins to pack on, primarily in the stomach, hips, thighs, and buttocks. This weight often stubbornly hangs around even in the face of changed eating patterns, increased exercise, and various other traditional methods of weight loss. Some may experience a small percentage of pounds lost, but overall, many will find that the weight is stubborn. Others may be able to lose weight easily, but find that if they deviate from a strict eating and exercise pattern that they quickly gain the weight back, plus some.

For most patients with Hashimoto's, once the disease is addressed, weight often begins to come off. For others who have high levels of systemic inflammation, even after hormone replacement and lifestyle changes, it can take weeks, months, or even years to see body weight reach desired levels. Remember that autoimmunity isn't a single-layered issue. It is multifaceted, and even when the major aggravating factors are addressed, tissues take time to become less inflamed, hormones take time to settle, and related conditions must be addressed individually.

Sleep Disorders and Insomnia

A common pattern associated with Hashimoto's is fatigue, along with bouts of insomnia or frequent night wakings. It seems illogical that when you're excessively tired your body won't let you sleep uninterrupted, but again, this is a result of the systemic nature of Hashimoto's. Many resort to over-the-counter or even prescribed sleep aids in the quest for sleep, but these often work for a while and then eventually lose their potency. Alternatively, sleep aids for some with thyroid disease may produce an almost opposite effect, or may have no effect whatsoever.

While sleep disorders and insomnia can be completely separate issues in and of themselves, many patients will find that their sleep, both quantity and quality, dramatically improves as Hashimoto's is treated and addressed with lifestyle and dietary changes. In fact, sleep quality as well as frequency of night wakings can become a barometer of sorts for the state of the thyroid. Hashimoto's patients may find that if night wakings return, their hormone replacement levels need to be tweaked, or other adjustments made.

Infertility and Recurrent Miscarriage

According to statistics cited in *Thyroid Healthy* by Suzy Cohen, RPh, more than 6.1 million women are impacted by infertility. Whether infertility is caused by Hashimoto's, whether it is one of several factors, or whether it is sparked during pregnancy, thyroid issues can wreak havoc on a woman's ability to conceive, stay pregnant, and recover well in the postpartum period. It is not common for women trying to conceive or those who become pregnant to be screened with anything more than TSH; however, many in the holistic and integrative communities believe that to properly practice preventive prenatal care, women should be screened before, during, and after pregnancy with the following tests:

- Free T3
- Free T4
- Reverse T3
- Thyroid antibodies

Because this disease affects women substantially more than men, and because hormone factors can trigger it (arguably none greater than pregnancy), it should become routine for women in their twenties and thirties to be monitored. Doing so could reduce the number of people who end up developing organ damage from months or years of antibody production that goes undetected.

If a woman who has Hashimoto's does become pregnant, it's imperative to properly monitor and treat the thyroid. When autoimmune thyroid disease is not effectively controlled during pregnancy, any of the following can result:

- Preeclampsia
- Anemia
- Placental abruption
- Postpartum hemorrhage
- Miscarriage
- Stillbirth
- Preterm birth
- Low birth weight
- Birth defects, including brain development disorders and neural tube defects
- Infant thyroid disorders
- Postpartum depression
- Postpartum anxiety
- Postpartum psychosis
- Inability to lose postpartum weight

QUESTION

How can I advocate for myself as a pregnant patient with Hashimoto's?
Finding an OB-GYN who is familiar with Hashimoto's and other auto-immune diseases is a start. Secondly, as long as your insurance will cover extra testing (be sure to check first), most OBs will be flexible about adding extra monitoring, especially with a history of autoimmunity and thyroid disease—which in most cases will mean a high-risk pregnancy. This can result in extra lab work, more ultrasounds, and fetal nonstress tests and growth scans as the pregnancy progresses.

Unfortunately, many women with undiagnosed thyroid disease may be able to conceive, but could have repeated, early pregnancy losses. Even women with diagnosed and controlled Hashimoto's have a greater likelihood of experiencing infertility or miscarriage, most likely due to potentially linked autoimmune disorders that are not controlled or diagnosed.

Hormonal Imbalance

Apart from fertility or pregnancy issues, thyroid disease can also contribute to generalized female hormone imbalances by exacerbating problems of low progesterone or estrogen dominance. These conditions can be associated with infertility or pregnancy problems, but they are also associated with PMS and mood disorders such as depression and anxiety. At one time, a study was conducted that tried to show that PMS is strictly related to hypothyroidism, but the protocol involved too much of an aggressive approach to hormone replacement and so the study was discredited. While it may not be proven that PMS is only a thyroid issue, it is certainly true that most women with Hashimoto's experience worse PMS, hormonal imbalances, and mood swings than women who do not have thyroid disease. Dr. Christiane Northrup links thyroid issues with estrogen dominance and progesterone deficiency because of a protein in the blood known as thyroid-binding globulin. This protein, as the name describes, actually binds thyroid hormone in the blood and reduces the amount available to be used by cells. The result is lowered thyroid function during this phase of the menstrual cycle, and it happens to be during the luteal phase, when progesterone should be higher. In cases of reduced progesterone and estrogen dominance, the give-and-take that is meant to happen with these two dominant female reproductive hormones does not happen. Estrogen continues to be dominant, and associated symptoms are often classed as PMS, when in fact they're the result of both excess estrogen and inadequate levels of thyroid hormone. Symptoms of estrogen dominance can include:

- Sleep difficulties or insomnia
- Fatigue
- Foggy thinking and confusion
- Slowed metabolism

- Reduced thyroid function
- Hair loss
- Weight gain, especially around stomach, hips, thighs, and buttocks
- Mood swings, especially depression, irritability, and anxiety
- Headaches
- Fibrocystic breasts
- Breast tenderness
- Breast swelling
- Bloating
- Irregular or extremely heavy menstrual periods
- Reduced libido

Because of the way that hormones overlap and play off of each other, it is rarely simple enough to blame hormone imbalances or disorders on one hormone alone. Hashimoto's may be the primary diagnosis, but as a result, estrogen dominance can occur. Treating thyroid disease may alleviate many hormone imbalances, but it may also be necessary to treat other hormone issues besides the thyroid.

Mood Disorders and Depression

Much research in the last few years has centered on vitamin D, particularly its hormone component. Since vitamin D can be synthesized in the human body as a result of direct sunlight activating the precursor form of the vitamin from cholesterol, it is considered a nutrient as well as a hormone. Vitamin D deficiency has been associated with a plethora of unpleasant disorders and symptoms, including mood disorders, depression, anxiety, chronic illness, and autoimmune disease—including Hashimoto's.

The Vitamin D Council reported on a study done by Dr. Nujen Bozkurt of Ankara University School of Medicine in Turkey, which monitored vitamin D levels in two groups of 180 Hashimoto's patients and one group of 180 controls, and discovered that almost 50 percent of Hashimoto's patients had critically low vitamin D levels. Current recommendations are not sufficient according to the Vitamin D Council, which recommends that adults get somewhere between 5,000 and 10,000 IU of vitamin D daily. Exposure to the sun can produce between 10,000 and 25,000 IU in anywhere from a few minutes to a few hours, but supplemental levels should not exceed 10,000 IU daily unless supervised by a doctor. Infants, children, and younger adults have fewer requirements. The standard lab range for adults is just 20–30 ng/mL, but integrative practitioners believe that optimal levels are closer to 50–70 ng/mL.

Moreover, the Bozkurt study found a direct relation between vitamin D levels and thyroid antibody levels. The higher the vitamin D was, the lower the antibodies were, and vice versa. The study also speculated that perhaps there is a relation between the severity of vitamin D deficiency and the progression of Hashimoto's, especially the amount of damage done to the thyroid by antibody attacks.

FACT

Most people know that vitamin D is produced in the body when skin is directly exposed to the sun, but wearing sunscreen negates this effect. Only slight exposure is needed, however, so it is essential to use sunscreen if you will be exposed long enough for your skin to turn pink or to burn. Vitamin D is produced long before the skin turns pink. Additionally, vitamin D synthesis does *not* take place from exposure to sunlight through a window.

So what comes first, the D deficiency, the mood disorder, or the thyroid disease? Or is it a perfect storm of all the above? Perhaps at the base is a genetic predisposition to thyroid disease and other conditions, and when vitamin D amounts dip below a healthy level, mechanisms get triggered (along with other environmental, lifestyle, and disease factors) that ignite inflammatory and autoimmune attacks within the body.

Celiac Disease

Celiac disease is an autoimmune condition where the intake of gluten mobilizes the immune system to mount an attack against the small intestine. This attack damages the villi, which are finger-like projections that are responsible for nutrient absorption. Current estimates suggest that 1 in every 100 people has celiac disease, and many more are likely undiagnosed since the symptoms can be vague or attributable to other conditions. Such symptoms include:

- Digestive upset
- Abdominal bloating
- Chronic widespread pain or localized abdominal pain
- Diarrhea
- Vomiting
- Unintentional weight loss
- Foul-smelling stool
- Fatigue
- Depression and mood swings
- Anxiety and panic attacks
- Menstrual abnormalities
- Tingling or numbness in extremities
- Canker sores
- Itchy skin or rashes
- Eczema

Because celiac disease is essentially ground zero for leaky gut formation (although other food allergies or toxins can trigger intestinal permeability, too), patients who have Hashimoto's should be tested for celiac disease or non-celiac gluten sensitivity. Regardless of whether a thyroid patient is found to be allergic or sensitive to gluten, she should avoid this inflammatory food because when broken down to the protein level, it resembles thyroid tissue. If your gut isn't perfectly closed—and most people have some level of leaky gut—these proteins enter the bloodstream and trigger autoimmune reactivity against the thyroid, or even system-wide, even if you are taking hormone replacement to "fix" your thyroid disease. Hashimoto's, celiac, and other chronic conditions are rarely so easily resolved. Dietary changes are vital in the journey of healing.

ALERT

Celiac disease is difficult to diagnose unless gluten is present in the body at the time of diagnosis. If you've already been living a gluten-free lifestyle because you have a family history of celiac, or because you know that it triggers autoimmune reactions with Hashimoto's, then it's not worth it to reintroduce gluten just to be told that it's bad for you. Adopting a gluten-free lifestyle for non-celiac reasons is a health-supportive decision that doesn't need a medical diagnosis to back it up.

Inflammatory and Digestive Disorders

Inflammatory bowel disease, or IBD, describes a group of chronic digestive conditions that impact the intestines and the colon. Three of the most commonly known are Crohn's disease, ulcerative colitis, and irritable bowel syndrome (IBS). With Crohn's disease, the GI tract, and primarily the small intestine, becomes inflamed. Ulcerative colitis is inflammation of the colon's top layer. These conditions have major symptoms in common, such as diarrhea, intestinal cramping, and sometimes bleeding. IBS is more vague—often a blanket term given to intestinal disorders that are distinctly not Crohn's or ulcerative colitis—but is a chronic disorder that involves symptoms such as constipation or diarrhea, bloating, and abdominal pain.

Inflammatory digestive disorders have a strong relation with autoimmunity, and it is common to find one or more present in men or women who have other presenting autoimmune conditions. Additionally, nearly a quarter of people who have one or more bowel disorders also have an immediate relative who also has a similar condition. That is highly indicative of genetic predisposition, which can certainly include immune reactivity.

The specific relation of Hashimoto's to inflammatory digestive disorders is linked to problems with nutrient absorption, specifically selenium. Selenium is a mineral that functions as an antioxidant, and it is also required for synthesis of thyroid hormone. When digestive or bowel disorders are present, selenium is one of the first minerals to be used up. Without a selenium-rich diet or supplementation, thyroid disorders will worsen. A study published in the *Journal of Rheumatology* even linked thyroid antibody reduction with improved selenium intakes.

Fibromyalgia

Fibromyalgia is a chronic pain disorder that is characterized by musculoskeletal pain that is typically evenly dispersed across the body, as well as joint aches, sleep disturbance, and excessive fatigue. The symptom overlap between Hashimoto's and fibromyalgia is uncanny, and often, one can be mistakenly diagnosed as the other. It is not uncommon, however, to find patients who have both conditions. Dr. Kenneth Blanchard, in his book *The Functional Approach to Hypothyroidism*, notes that even when he had patients who did not have thyroid disease according to lab results, he often prescribed thyroid medication to those who appeared to have fibromyalgia. Most of them felt enough of an improvement after starting thyroid hormone replacement that they wanted to continue, even if it was not a complete cure.

Although the mechanism isn't fully understood, it is quite common for patients who have autoimmune thyroid disease to also have fibromyalgia, or to eventually develop it. Rheumatoid arthritis can be included here, as it is also an autoimmune condition that involves widespread pain and inflammation, and which can also often be misdiagnosed as fibromyalgia or Hashimoto's. Symptoms of fibromyalgia and rheumatoid arthritis often improve based on lifestyle factors, such as diet, exercise, and other restorative therapies. Weather, too, can have an impact on pain levels for those who have these body-wide conditions, often improving in warm, dry weather, and worsening in cool, damp weather. Thyroid disease, of course, has temperature associations, as decreased thyroid function can make you much more sensitive to cold.

Mononucleosis and Epstein-Barr

There are numerous viral infections that can cause systemic or long-term problems, but perhaps the most well known are mononucleosis and the virus that typically causes it, Epstein-Barr Virus (EBV). Research by the Department of Pathology at Comenius University in the Slovak Republic identified a high prevalence of Hashimoto's and EBV together, implying that EBV may have a role in triggering autoimmune thyroid disease as a prevailing environmental factor.

A different slice of the EBV-Hashimoto's puzzle is considered by Dr. Nikolas R. Hedberg, who in an article on the website HypothyroidMom.com posits EBV to be a cause of Hashimoto's due to something known as molecular mimicry. Basically, a viral infection enters the body, but due to specific genetic absence of immune cells, the virus remains quietly active long after the primary infection. The immune system continues to fight the virus, and in the process of overactivation, the immune system mistakenly views organ tissue as components of the virus and attacks. As long as the infection remains active within the body, the autoimmune fight against the organ will persist. Dr. Hedberg notes specifically that people who have Hashimoto's are missing an immune cell that controls EBV, and that this is why the virus is able to remain active for so long.

How do I know if I have EBV or another chronic or hidden viral infection?
Almost all viral infections can be tested via blood work, and viral titers will be present in both current, active infections, as well as dormant infections that could still be problematic. The key is not necessarily to look for signs of new or primary infection, but rather to assess whether or not the mere presence of the virus could be enough to trigger autoimmune reactivity.

Whether Hashimoto's came first or was triggered as a result of a chronic viral infection, it is essential to be screened for these during the investigative process. Not only is EBV associated with Hashimoto's, but several other viral infections can be as well, including cytomegalovirus, parvovirus, and even various strains of influenza. Even if they aren't environmental triggers or stealth causes of Hashimoto's, the presence of autoimmunity and leaky gut can leave the body vulnerable to viral infections that can become chronic in a body that is already weakened from self-attack.

Other Chronic Conditions

This chapter does not list every potential condition associated with Hashimoto's, and there are easily dozens more: multiple sclerosis, Sjögren's syndrome, systemic lupus erythematosus, Lyme disease, sclerosis, and dermatitis herpetiformis, to name a few. Once the body is left defenseless from the attack of its own immune system, genetic susceptibility will determine what organs and body systems will become impacted by continued and spreading antibody production.

The good news is that autoimmune reactivity can be lessened through various lifestyle, medical, and natural treatments and interventions, and while there is no cure for many autoimmune disorders, the possibility of remission is quite real. Many have fully eliminated symptoms of Hashimoto's and other autoimmune conditions by maintaining a lifestyle that is support-ive to their various weakened organs, and to the digestive system as a whole.

Healing is a relative term when it comes to time frames and specific results, since bioindividuality has a lot to do with how rapidly you will respond to treatment, specific medications, and dietary changes. Even the climate and environment that you live in can have an impact on both your genetics and your immune system, which will definitely affect how quickly and how well your body adapts and responds. Thankfully, in an age of research and integrative medicine that bridges gaps between conventional and holistic approaches, there is a healing path to be found for everyone, if you know where to look.

CHAPTER 3

How to Heal Thyroid Disease

While there is currently no known method for preventing the onset of Hashimoto's thyroiditis, there are certainly a number of ways to treat it, heal the body, and move the disease into remission. As research continues to delve deeper into the immune system, the microbiome, and the way that whole body systems communicate with each other, as well as genetic health and environmental triggers, perhaps there will a come a day when preventive measures can be taken to avoid destruction of the thyroid gland or to address the disease before it progresses into full-blown autoimmunity. Until then, there is a vast framework of conventional, complementary, and nutritional therapies that can move your body into a state of restored and renewed health.

Autoimmunity Is More Than a Single Organ

The process of healing thyroid disease is so much bigger than "fixing" the thyroid. But it can be a natural assumption that if you start on thyroid medication that all the symptoms will go away. As you will see in this chapter, this is simply not the case. Not only is there the process of determining which thyroid hormone replacement to use (there are several options, including synthetic and natural), there is also the issue of deciding if any additional conditions need to be treated. Aggravating lifestyle factors also need to be eliminated, while therapeutic behaviors need to be added. Dietary changes need to take place that will have systemic benefits, not just for the thyroid, but for the digestive system, the gut, the immune system, and widespread inflammation.

ALERT

According to a 2010 study in *Maedica: A Journal of Clinical Medicine*, approximately 25 percent of people with one autoimmune disorder will develop additional autoimmune diseases. When a patient has three or more concurrent autoimmune disorders, it is known as multiple autoimmune syndrome (MAS). While it is not yet fully understood why some people are more prone to developing several disorders, genetic predisposition and family history seem to play a role. People at risk for developing MAS are those who already have one autoimmune disorder or who have immediate family members with one or more autoimmune diseases.

Healing autoimmunity and eventually reaching a state of remission is not a one-step process. It does not happen as the result of a single prescription, and it generally involves much more than just the thyroid. After all, autoimmune disease isn't caused by a single organ. It begins as a cascade of events that set off a chain reaction of auto-aggression. When this happens, the immune system is impacted, along with the digestive tract, the brain, the heart, the liver, and perhaps other organs. Autoimmune disorders are complex, and Hashimoto's is no exception. Environmental triggers, genetic predisposition, food allergies, nutrient deficiencies, hormone imbalances, and inflammation can be just some of the many factors that need to be considered and potentially addressed.

What to Expect from Conventional Treatment

Conventional or traditional medical treatment for Hashimoto's disease can vary in the sense that some doctors won't recognize Hashimoto's initially, leaving patients confused and without a proper diagnosis. In other cases, doctors may misdiagnose Hashimoto's as fibromyalgia or as depression, and prescribe pain medication or antidepressants, but not thyroid medication. This can be hit or miss in providing relief. Some patients may feel temporarily better if they happen to have those conditions in addition to Hashimoto's, but in most cases, many will still feel unwell, fatigued, and will present with various other symptoms of hypothyroidism.

In the event that doctors do diagnose Hashimoto's thyroiditis, the most conventional medical approach is hormone replacement and little else.

Prescriptions

The typical prescription for Hashimoto's is levothyroxine, which is synthetic T4. This medication is sold as Synthroid or Levoxyl. Some patients respond well to this treatment, but others have difficulty converting the T4 into usable, active T3, and so an alternative is to prescribe a synthetic T3 (Cytomel) in addition to the T4, or to use a medication that combines both hormones, such as Thyrolar.

Some physicians will also employ a prescription that contains some glandular hormone, typically from porcine sources. The most popular of these "natural" prescriptions is Armour Thyroid. Some patients who do not respond well or at all to levothyroxine respond better to natural desiccated thyroid (NDT) sources.

Absorption Factors

Some thyroid medications, especially synthetic versions, are particularly susceptible to absorption problems. They typically need to be taken without food, particularly food sources that can block or interfere with metabolizing them. These sources can include coffee, iron-containing foods, soy products, and grapefruit juice. Most doctors recommend taking thyroid prescriptions first thing in the morning, at least half an hour before breakfast or coffee, at the same time every day. NDT is less susceptible to absorption issues, and while it should still be taken at the same time each day, it can typically be consumed with food.

Will I have to take thyroid medication for the rest of my life?
The answer to this largely depends on how long you have had Hashimoto's, how much damage has been done to your thyroid, and how many other autoimmune or chronic disorders you have. Many conventional practitioners will tell you that hormone replacement is a lifelong thing. More holistic practitioners may offer some hope of reducing or eliminating thyroid medication at some point, but again, this is still largely determinant on the amount of damage that the antibodies have done to your thyroid.

Alternative, Integrative, and Holistic Therapies

Hashimoto's is more frequently embraced by practitioners who employ alternative, integrative, and holistic health practices. These can include integrative medical doctors, naturopaths, nutritionists, or chiropractors. While more natural-minded practitioners may more readily acknowledge and address Hashimoto's, it is important to consider their qualifications and experience in working with thyroid disorders. Autoimmune disease is a complex health problem that can be dramatically worsened by certain ill-informed protocols and by practitioners who are not well versed in the subject. Learning to ask the right questions of your practitioners will be vital to your ability to heal.

Questions to Ask Alternative Practitioners

When interviewing potential practitioners, be sure to ask the following questions:

1. What experience do you have with Hashimoto's thyroiditis? How do you diagnose it?
2. What is a standard treatment protocol that you use for Hashimoto's?

3. What success have you had with patients who have had Hashimoto's disease?
4. How do you address autoimmunity and leaky gut?
5. What should I expect from seeking treatment with you?

Use the information contained in this book to gauge your sense of confidence in the practitioner's replies. Being able to freely communicate with the practitioner who is monitoring and treating your Hashimoto's is key because sometimes the only thing you have to go on is how you are feeling. Lab tests may not always be fully reflective of progress, and a truly skilled practitioner will be able to use your description of how you're feeling and the status of your symptoms to further investigate.

Common Alternative and Integrative Approaches

Autoimmune disease is in the best hands when in the care of practitioners who blend alternative and integrative therapies with traditional medical approaches. Integrative medicine blends both worlds, utilizing holistic nutrition principles, supplementation, and milder forms of treatment when possible before resorting to prescription medication. It does, however, acknowledge that there is a time and a place for conventional pharmaceutical therapy. Unlike some natural practitioners who are resistant to any form of prescription drug, integrative and functional medical and nutritionally minded professionals take into account the big picture of what is happening within the body and then come up with a plan to restore balance within the body. Conditions are not assessed individually, but rather, as a collective problem that needs to be addressed, one layer at a time. Layers that don't make sense are not dismissed or covered over with medication, but instead are further explored, often resulting in multiple diagnoses that present a more complete picture of the current state of a patient's health.

Integrative and functional medicine view Hashimoto's as a multifaceted disease that requires a full-throttle approach. Simply replacing thyroid hormone will not do the trick. While further investigation will be done to root out the cause of the disease, other supplements and lifestyle support will be given to help bring balance as quickly as possible. Some common herbs and supplements that are used to address Hashimoto's include the following:

- **Ashwagandha:** An adaptogenic herb that supports the adrenal glands by reducing the stress response. It is beneficial for Hashimoto's patients because it can help with T4 to T3 conversion.
- **L-tyrosine:** An amino acid that assists in the production of thyroid hormone, it increases effectiveness of thyroid medication or the body's natural thyroid hormone production. Dosage adjustments may need to be made to hormone replacement medication since L-tyrosine could reduce the amount needed to produce balanced hormone levels.
- **Natural desiccated thyroid supplements:** Similar to NDT thyroid medication, supplement versions exist that may also contain other thyroid-supportive nutrients. Sometimes these products are available at health food stores, but most of them may only be available through professional supplement lines acquired from nutritionists, naturopathic doctors, or chiropractors.
- **Selenium:** A trace mineral required for conversion of T4 to T3, selenium also acts as an antioxidant within the body.
- **Vitamin A:** A fat-soluble vitamin that helps the thyroid produce T4, usually only deficient in people who do not eat animal products.
- **Zinc:** A mineral that helps convert T4 to T3 and supports general immune wellness.
- **Iron:** A mineral required for healthy red blood cells and hemoglobin levels, it is also associated with thyroid hormone production.
- **Seaweed:** A natural source of iodine, seaweed as a supplement is considered a safer form of iodine supplementation for Hashimoto's patients, since direct iodine supplementation with the presence of autoimmunity is controversial. In some cases direct iodine supplementation can increase antibody production and worsen Hashimoto's. Iodine, however, is essential for thyroid hormone production.
- **EFAs:** Essential fatty acids are beneficial for thyroid health because they increase energy levels in the cells of the thyroid, vital for an organ depressed from immune attacks.
- **Bioidentical compounded progesterone:** Different from progesterone creams, this is a medical prescription that is often utilized by integrative practitioners. Since thyroid dysfunction can suppress progesterone production, and estrogen dominance can worsen thyroid symptoms, taking bioidentical progesterone during the luteal phase of a woman's

cycle can help create balance to reproductive hormones and decrease unpleasant thyroid symptoms such as PMS, anxiety, mood disorders, and bloating.

- **Vitamin D$_3$:** Essential for immune health, mood balance, and autoimmune recovery, the sunshine vitamin is fat-soluble and can be stored in cells, but most people are still deficient. People should be tested prior to starting high-dose supplementation since toxicity is possible. If levels are low (below 50 ng/mL), 10,000 IU daily can help restore balance. If levels are higher than 50 ng/mL, 5,000 IU daily is a good maintenance dosage.

- **Nux vomica:** A homeopathic drug that eases unpleasant thyroid symptoms such as fatigue, sensitivity to cold, irritability, and constipation, this is not a replacement for thyroid hormone medication, but rather a stop-gap to help decrease symptoms in the interim between starting treatment and awaiting results.

- **B-complex:** The B vitamin family are often supplemented in complex form because they play off of each other, and are most effective when given at the same time. A deficiency of B$_2$ can depress overall endocrine function, while B$_3$ aids cells in receiving and delivering energy. B$_6$ has a role in converting iodine to thyroid hormone, while B$_{12}$ needs to be replenished because low thyroid function makes it less absorbable from dietary sources. Insufficient levels of B$_{12}$ can result in pernicious anemia, which can contribute to fatigue and several other symptoms associated with Hashimoto's.

- **Copper:** A trace mineral only required in tiny doses, it gets displaced in the wake of zinc supplementation, so it should be added to a supplement protocol to maintain balance.

- **Magnesium:** A mineral that is associated with muscle relaxation, it is beneficial in Hashimoto's for increased energy production at the cellular level. It also helps relieve common muscular and joint aches and pains that are often felt by those who have Hashimoto's.

- **Evening primrose oil:** An essential fatty acid that helps to restore vitality to skin and hair, both of which are often affected by Hashimoto's disease.

- **Maca:** An herb that can help create balance throughout the entire endocrine system, and may help reduce dosages for thyroid hormone replacement after regular use.

- **Glutamine:** An amino acid required for proper immune function and a healthy intestinal wall, often found to be deficient in patients with Hashimoto's.
- **Alkaline phosphatase:** An enzyme associated with the gut's ability to detoxify and reduce reaction to gram-negative intestinal bacteria that can overpower gram-positive or "good" bacteria, resulting in infections, autoimmunity, and leaky gut. Alkaline phosphatase deficiency is associated with systemic inflammation and autoimmune reactivity, and can commonly be seen in Hashimoto's patients. Alkaline phosphatase can be increased within the intestinal tract by consuming fermented foods, grassfed butter, ginger, and black pepper.

Nutrition Therapy

In a true whole-food program like the Paleo diet, it is optimal for all essential nutrients to be obtained from food sources alone. This can be achieved by people who do not have chronic health issues, and in some cases, by people who do have certain health conditions. In cases of autoimmunity, however, because of gut issues like malabsorption as well as long-term nutrient deficiencies, it can be necessary to supplement specific nutrients. Supplementation may be short or long in duration, but beyond a basic multivitamin, rarely is it permanent. As autoimmunity is addressed, antibodies decrease, and as the intestinal wall heals from leaky gut, additional nutrient supplementation will become less critical.

The principles of nutrition therapy are that food is medicine, and that the right combination of food can meet the body's nutritional needs. As such, nutrient supplementation should be just that: supplemental. Vitamins and herbs should not be taken to counteract poor dietary choices or habits, but rather, to enhance them and to speed the process of healing.

Paleo Diet and Nutrition Therapy

Hashimoto's and other autoimmune diseases respond very well to nutrition therapy, particularly when a Paleo diet is in play. Paleo naturally excludes foods that are damaging to the gut wall or that perpetuate autoimmune reactions. Additionally, dietary protocols aimed at helping to restore the body from thyroid disease will be rich in good-quality fats and abundant in vegetables. Regular intake of quality-sourced protein is also essential, as well as other nutrients found in fruit, nuts, and seeds.

Patients with Hashimoto's generally do not benefit from low-carb diets since carbohydrates are required for energy production. Switching to a ketogenic diet can often produce more unpleasant symptoms and create more of a body burden for those already sick with autoimmune disorders unless some healing has already taken place. Balance and support are of primary importance when beginning a nutritionally supportive Paleo program for Hashimoto's. You aren't aiming for extreme weight loss, instant transformations, or wacky food combinations. You're aiming to replenish nutrient deficiencies, to restore proper digestive and gut health, and to replace antagonistic foods with supportive ones.

Methylation and Genetic Health

The term *methylation* has become quite popular in recent years thanks to the wider availability of genetic testing. Methylation refers to a biochemical act of combining one carbon with three hydrogens (a methyl group) and applying it to body processes that are vital for life. Methylation can turn your genes on and off, boost immunity to fight infections, and help detox the body of toxins and chemical invaders. It is also required for clear thinking, DNA repair, and multiple other body functions.

ESSENTIAL

Methylation and MTHFR is an emerging topic of popularity in the integrative medicine world. The defect is so common that as many as 1 out of every 2 people have a certain level of MTHFR genetic mutations to contend with. Dr. Benjamin Lynch, a naturopathic doctor, is the country's leading expert on MTHFR and methylation issues. You can find an endless supply of information on the subject at his website, MTHFR.net, as well as read specifically how MTHFR and thyroid are related in the chapter he authored from the book *Stop the Thyroid Madness II*.

MTHFR is most commonly associated with methylation, and is a gene that produces an enzyme, also known as MTHFR, or by its full name: methylenetetrahydrofolate reductase (and that is precisely why it is abbreviated). Some refer to it as the "mother father" gene, since it is inherited from both parents, and the genetic mutations that they carry will determine the ones that you have.

The MTHFR gene is present in all the body's cells, and its primary focus is to convert folate to the biologically active form of methylfolate. When the MTHFR gene is mutated, it does not function effectively, and MTHFR enzyme production is inhibited. This results in deficiency or inadequate levels of methylfolate. Some doctors test for MTHFR in conjunction with thyroid disease, or with associated conditions of thyroid disease such as infertility or recurrent pregnancy loss. Unfortunately, the conventional medical approach to MTHFR genetic mutations is to prescribe high-dose folic acid. Folic acid is the synthetic form of folate and must go through conversions within the body to become the bioavailable methyl form. If you have an MTHFR mutation, regardless of how much folic acid you pump your body full of, you will still likely suffer the effects of methylfolate deficiency. The issue is not a lack of folic acid, but rather a lack of conversion enzyme. In order to address MTHFR properly, the type of folate supplemented should be one that does not require biological conversion to be activated. For most people who have MTHFR mutations, this means taking activated methylfolate along with activated B_{12} directly. Folate and B_{12} require each other to function, and a deficiency of one will result in problems with the other. Many supplement formulations provide not only the active forms of B_{12} and folate, but also the other vitamins in the B complex family.

MTHFR, Folate, and Hashimoto's

So what do MTHFR and folate have to do with Hashimoto's disease or thyroid issues? Symptoms associated with reduced MTHFR genetic function and associated low or deficient levels of methylfolate include many overlapping symptoms or conditions with thyroid disease:

- Anxiety
- Depression
- Sleep disorders and insomnia
- Skin disorders

- Chronic fatigue
- Neurological disorders
- Autism
- Cardiovascular disorders or disease
- Cancer

Supplementing with methylfolate does not fix the issue of having an MTHFR mutation or having thyroid disease, but it can be a major step in the process of healing. It is essential to get tested since there are a few combinations of MTHFR genetic mutations that can impact the level of supplementation that you may require. Two specific genes are tested for: MTHFR C677T and MTHFR A1298C. Of these, you can carry one or two copies. Your parents each have two copies, and you receive one copy from each of them, giving you two copies. Of your two copies, you would pass one on to your child, and your child would receive one from your spouse or partner.

When a parent is a carrier of two mutated versions (homozygous) of an MTHFR gene, she will definitely pass on one mutated copy to any children. When both parents are homozygous, the child will definitely carry two genetic mutations. The three potential combinations for greater MTHFR dysfunction and methylfolate deficiency are:

- Homozygous for MTHFR A1298C
- Homozygous for MTHFR C677T
- Compound heterozygous with one A1298C mutation and one C677T

Of course, you can also carry a single heterozygous mutation of either and still have a slight risk for low folate levels, but the deficiency risk is significantly increased when two mutated genes are present.

The subject of correcting and balancing methylation is more appropriate for an entire library of books and is well beyond the scope of this one. More resources on the subject can be found in Appendix B.

Addressing Inflammation

Not only do autoimmune attacks fuel inflammatory responses in a circular relationship that also involves inflammation perpetuating autoimmune attacks, but methylfolate deficiency can also contribute to systemic inflammation in the form of elevated homocysteine levels and other inflammation markers like C-reactive protein, fibrinogen, and white blood cells.

Addressing systemic inflammation in Hashimoto's disease is not as simple as taking supplemental methylfolate, although that can be a beneficial factor in some cases. Autoimmune disease is a multifaceted condition that can never be treated by a single-pronged approach. The same is true for inflammation—there is rarely a single cause, but rather, a cascade of varying factors that must all be addressed simultaneously to help produce a cooling effect within the body.

Factors associated with the reduction of inflammation in autoimmune thyroid disease include the following:

- **Methylfolate and methyl-B$_{12}$ supplementation:** As has already been discussed.
- **Optimizing vitamin D$_3$ levels:** A study from *JAMA Internal Medicine* reported that as many as 75 percent of Americans do not get enough vitamin D. Other research links increased levels of inflammatory markers with decreased levels of the sunshine vitamin. The vitamin undoubtedly has a role in disease prevention as well as in healing. Optimizing vitamin D levels can have a systemic effect on reducing the body's inflammatory load.
- **Antioxidant protection:** Eating a diet rich in fresh vegetables and fruit is associated with lower levels of inflammatory markers, and by following a Paleo diet, the body will receive therapeutic nutrients for healing.

The Stress Connection

Reducing inflammation cannot take place without the simultaneous and perpetual reduction of stress, including physical, mental, and emotional stress. While stress alone is not enough to make you sick, it can trigger a cascade effect of inflammatory processes that can trigger genetic tendencies in association with lifestyle and environmental factors to produce and perpetuate autoimmune reactivity. You can do all the right things physically, but if your life is still stressing you out on a regular basis, your body will have a hard time focusing on recovery and repair, and may take much longer to achieve remission.

Stress is closely tied to both digestive issues, including leaky gut, and thyroid disorders. But whether stress worsens as a result of these physical issues or whether it worsens the physical issues is a point that isn't necessarily worth arguing. Any health-promoting lifestyle should focus on reducing all sources of stress.

Food Allergy and Sensitivity

In order for the body to heal from Hashimoto's, offending foods that trigger leaky gut reactions and the subsequent organ attacks need to be removed. Gluten and dairy are the most common food triggers, but several other foods can be cross-reactive to those, including oats, rice, and soy. Because the Paleo diet eliminates all forms of grains and legumes, people with Hashimoto's often thrive on it, although it isn't always understood that this is the reasoning behind it. A Paleo food plan will also be richer in protein than the average American diet, and since protein is required for thyroid hormone production, this too becomes a therapeutic answer to thyroid disease.

While following a strict Paleo diet can often be enough to achieve healing from Hashimoto's, some patients prefer to see on paper what food sensitivities or other allergies they have. Numerous labs exist to test food allergy and sensitivity; however, many medical and nutrition professionals have their doubts about the complete accuracy of these results.

Implementing an elimination diet within the Paleo diet can also be a useful tool in assessing specific allergens or intolerances. More information on this can be found in Appendix B.

How Leaky Gut Causes Autoimmunity

It has been established that leaky gut can contribute to autoimmune reactivity by allowing undigested proteins to circulate within the bloodstream, activating the immune system and increasing inflammation. Healing leaky gut is critical to treatment of Hashimoto's thyroiditis and all other autoimmune conditions.

The principles outlined in this chapter will go a long way toward addressing leaky gut, but some additional antioxidants may be helpful in restoring proper barrier function to the gut, and in decreasing overall inflammation levels. These include:

- **L-carnitine:** An amino acid required for energy production as well as antioxidant production from the oxidative results of energy production.
- **Coenzyme Q-10:** An antioxidant vital for proper cell function, energy production, and tissue maintenance.
- **Curcumin:** A chemical compound found in turmeric associated with reduced inflammation.
- **Quercetin:** A flavonoid antioxidant that combats free radical damage, inflammation, and natural processes of aging.

How an Unbalanced Microbiome Contributes to Autoimmunity

Last but not least in a healing plan for Hashimoto's are probiotics. In the initial phase of resetting the gut and attempting to down-regulate the immune system's attacks on the thyroid gland as well as other organs, good bacteria needs to be replenished to combat the trillions of gram-negative bacteria that have taken up residence in the intestinal tract.

Gram-negative bacteria are the types of bacteria found in the gastrointestinal tract. They are often referred to as "bad" bacteria. One of the more well known kinds of gram-negative bacteria is *E. coli*. Gram-negative bacteria generally cause disease and infection when they outnumber and overpower the gram-positive, or "good," bacteria that the gut needs for balance. Gram-negative bacteria can quickly become strong enough to produce devastating consequences ranging from the historical outbreaks of cholera and the bubonic plague to modern instances of superbugs, antibiotic-resistant bacteria, and chronic autoimmunity, leaky gut, and infection.

At the heart of almost every autoimmune disease is intestinal permeability. Since the body is comprised of even more bacteria than cells, it is a sizable war to be waged. Probiotic supplements can be useful in addition to probiotic-rich foods. In the initial stages of healing Hashimoto's, as well as in the quest to achieve and maintain remission, high-dose probiotic supplementation may be beneficial, especially if antibiotic treatment has been used at any time in the past. Antibiotics destroy gram-positive bacteria, but gram-negative bacteria are increasingly able to resist and survive even after antibiotic treatment. It is not currently known how many CFUs (colony-forming units) of gram-positive, beneficial bacteria are required to displace even a single CFU of gram-negative bacteria. High-dose and broad probiotic strains don't necessarily immediately counteract the massive presence of gram-negative bacteria, but they can certainly be beneficial and have fewer consequences than broad, high-dose antibiotic treatment. Numerous strains of gram-negative bacteria have adapted to become antibiotic resistant, and so when they cannot be beaten, a holistic alternative is to outnumber them with beneficial bacteria.

Probiotics

Probiotic supplements have dramatically increased in popularity in recent years thanks to the emerging research on the microbiome, digestive and immune health, and leaky gut. Most health food stores will carry several varieties, and even big-box superstores and supermarkets now carry at least a few versions of probiotics. Product quality, however, can largely differ between brands, and it is essential to take a high-quality, pharmaceutical-grade supplement. Cheaper, poor-quality probiotics may contain fewer beneficial strains of bacteria, or may not contain as many live cultures as the packaging claims. Many shelf-stable probiotics (i.e., those that do not have to be refrigerated) claim to be as potent as refrigerated versions, but for cultures to remain live and active, they need to be kept in cool, dark environments—like that of the refrigerator and dark packaging. Probiotic supplements can be extremely expensive, but in most cases you get what you pay for. Investing in probiotic supplements at high doses for a short duration can have long-lasting impacts on the gut's restoration and the path toward remission.

Probiotic supplements come in a wide variety of strains, combinations, and dosages. Determining the specific strains and doses that will achieve the greatest impact on your gut health and autoimmunity should be left to a nutrition or integrative medical practitioner in order to get the best results from the protocol. Additionally, practitioners have often vetted brands for quality and consistency, and can offer insights on which provide good results and which might not be worth your time or money. Dose recommendations for Hashimoto's patients can range from a few million CFUs to several billion or even trillion. It all depends on the severity of your leaky gut and autoimmune symptoms, as well as your current digestive health.

Take a Multilayered Approach

By taking a multifaceted approach to Hashimoto's, including dietary changes, lifestyle adjustments, nutrient replenishment, leaky gut restoration, and more, not only are you working toward remission from a complicated autoimmune disorder, but you are also simultaneously addressing other chronic conditions that may be present. Additionally, you will be living a lifestyle that will naturally be preventive to the development of future additional chronic, autoimmune, and inflammatory diseases.

CHAPTER 4

What Is Paleo?

The Paleo diet has become quite popular in recent years, largely due to the success of low-carb food plans and frequent celebrity endorsements, not to mention emerging research that proves it leads to health improvements (including reduced body fat, lowered cholesterol, improved digestion, and a natural defense against cancer, diabetes, and heart disease). Also known as the caveman diet, Paleo (short for Paleolithic) emulates the clean-eating hunter-gatherer diet of our ancestors, favoring high-quality meats, fruit, vegetables, and seeds, and avoiding processed foods, grains, legumes, and dairy.

Principles of the Paleo Diet

If you're considering a switch to a Paleo diet, does that mean that you need to live in a cave, hunt your own game, and wear animal prints? Far from it! Living a Paleo lifestyle is about learning to adopt the same principles of eating that the cavemen lived by. While they had no choice in the matter, today you have the option of eating in just about any manner that you so desire. Unfortunately, the standard American diet has led to a widespread epidemic of heart disease, cancer, and type 2 diabetes, along with chronic digestive disorders, autoimmune disease like Hashimoto's, and obesity. Choosing to eat a Paleo diet is a major step toward investing in your health today and for the rest of your life.

The Paleo diet prioritizes foods that nourish the whole body, and avoids foods that cause digestive sluggishness and inflammation. The basics of eating Paleo include virtually any unprocessed meats, fats, vegetables, fruit, nuts, and seeds, which means that you definitely won't starve. It may require a major shift in your approach to food, but armed with a list of Paleo do's and don'ts, you'll master the concept in no time and be on your way to a richer, fuller way of living.

ESSENTIAL

Online shopping has revolutionized the Paleo world by making it more affordable and convenient than ever to find compatible foods. You can order Paleo staples such as coconut oil, ghee, canned wild-caught salmon, almond flour, and more from online retailers like Amazon, Thrive Market, Vitacost, and One Stop Paleo Shop.

In addition to the specific food categories that are not Paleo, the Paleo diet also avoids refined and processed foods. This means that you'll have to learn to read food labels and be much choosier about the quality of the food that you purchase. Thanks to the increased popularity of the Paleo diet, you can find Paleo-compliant foods at almost all supermarkets, health food stores, and even online.

Paleo is also all about eating locally sourced products, which is great for both you and your local economy. Purchasing farm-fresh eggs from the farmers' market or produce stand, along with vegetables, fruit, and meats, will provide you with the freshest ingredients and give you a personal connection to the food that you're putting into your body. This was what the cavemen did, out of necessity, but you can do it as a luxury. Of course, if you live in an area that is not equipped with a farmers' market, you can still reap the benefits of Paleo living by shopping at your grocery store or co-op.

What Paleo Is Not

As much as critics of Paleo love to hate on it, the Paleo diet is not a fad diet. There are no gimmicks or tricks—it's simply about eating whole foods that equip your body to function at its best. While Paleo often gets lumped into the low-carb diet fad, it actually doesn't have to be low-carb at all. One of the best features of the Paleo diet that few other food plans can claim is that it can be completely customized to your particular health goals and dietary needs. Paleo can be low- or high-carb, low- or high-calorie, and low- or high-maintenance. Even if you hate cooking, there is a way to make Paleo work for you.

Other critics of Paleo insist that it's too expensive and impractical to maintain. While you can certainly spend a small fortune on Paleo foods, with some smart decisions you can make Paleo work for any budget, large or small. It's also safe for the whole family, so by batch-cooking foods for everyone and not having to prepare two completely separate meal plans, you will save time and money.

FACT

Critics of Paleo insist that by eliminating dairy products, you won't get your recommended daily amount of calcium. One cup of milk contains 305 milligrams of calcium, but you can also get between 200 and 300 milligrams of calcium from the following: 1 cup of collard greens, 2 cups of kale, 1 (4-ounce) can of sardines, or 1 (6-ounce) can of wild-caught salmon.

Finally, the other major complaint against the Paleo diet is that you'll be missing out on key nutrients if you avoid entire categories of foods, like grains and dairy products. This is simply not true. Every nutrient necessary for total body wellness can be found in a well-balanced Paleo diet. Pasture-raised meats and free-range eggs are rich in protein, B vitamins, amino acids, and iron, while fruit, vegetables, nuts, and seeds contain a wide variety of fiber, minerals (including calcium), vitamins, and antioxidants. Healthy Paleo fats, such as coconut oil, ghee, salmon, and lard (yes, lard!), contain omega-3 and omega-6 fatty acids that support heart and brain health.

Foods to Eat and Foods to Avoid

Foods to eat on the Paleo diet include unprocessed meats, eggs, seafood, vegetables, fruit, nuts, seeds, fats, and natural sweeteners.

MEATS, EGGS, AND SEAFOOD
- Beef (including beef liver)
- Chicken (including chicken liver)
- Turkey
- Pork, ham, and bacon
- Bison
- Lamb
- Duck
- Deer (and other game meats)
- Eggs
- Salmon
- Sardines
- Halibut
- Shrimp (and other shellfish)
- Tuna
- Tilapia
- Cod
- Mackerel

VEGETABLES AND FRUIT
- Greens (arugula, beet greens, cabbage, bok choy, chard, collard greens, dandelion greens, kale, spinach, lettuce, romaine, radicchio, watercress)
- Cruciferous vegetables (broccoli, Brussels sprouts, cauliflower, artichokes)
- Root vegetables (turnips, white potatoes, sweet potatoes, asparagus, celery, garlic, kohlrabi, leeks, onions)
- Fruiting vegetables (avocados, bell peppers, cucumbers, eggplant, squash, sweet peppers, tomatillos, tomatoes, zucchini)

- Herbs (all kinds)
- Sea vegetables (all kinds)
- Berries (strawberries, blueberries, blackberries, raspberries, cranberries, grapes, bananas)
- Pit and core fruit (apricots, nectarines, peaches, cherries, plums, apples, pears)
- Citrus fruit (grapefruit, oranges, tangerines, limes, lemons, tangelos, kumquats)
- Melons (watermelon, cantaloupe, honeydew)
- Tropical fruit (figs, dates, mangoes, pineapples, coconut, passionfruit, pomegranates, kiwifruit, papaya)
- Rhubarb
- Star fruit

NUTS, SEEDS, AND FATS

- Almonds (including almond butter, almond flour)
- Brazil nuts
- Cashews (including cashew butter)
- Coconut (including oil, butter, aminos, milk, flesh, sap)
- Flaxseeds (including oil, whole, and ground)
- Hazelnuts (including hazelnut butter and flour)
- Macadamia nuts
- Olives (including olive oil)
- Pecans
- Pine nuts
- Pistachios
- Pumpkin seeds
- Sesame seeds (including oil)
- Sunflower seeds (including sunflower butter)
- Walnuts (including oil)
- Lard
- Tallow
- Ghee
- Duck fat
- Avocado oil
- Paleo mayonnaise

NATURAL SWEETENERS

- Raw honey
- Grade B maple syrup and maple sugar
- Coconut sugar and syrup
- Date sugar
- Stevia leaf
- Molasses

Foods that are not Paleo, and should be avoided, include dairy products, grains, legumes, beans, vegetable and hydrogenated oils, artificial flavors and sweeteners, and refined sugars and syrups. This is not a complete list, but gives you a good idea.

DAIRY PRODUCTS

- Milk
- Kefir and yogurt
- Sour cream
- Cream cheese
- Cheese
- Ice cream
- Butter (unless it is organic, grassfed butter)
- Half-and-half and creamer

GRAINS, LEGUMES, AND BEANS

- Wheat, barley, and rye
- White and brown rice
- Teff
- Sorghum
- Couscous
- Lentils
- All kinds of beans
- Peanuts
- Soybeans (and all soy products, including tofu and soy sauce)

VEGETABLE AND HYDROGENATED OILS

- Margarine
- Canola oil

- Soybean oil
- Corn oil
- Cottonseed oil
- Peanut oil

ARTIFICIAL AND REFINED FLAVORS AND SWEETENERS

- Sucralose
- Sugar alcohols (sorbitol, mannitol, xylitol, erythritol, maltitol, etc.)
- Dextrose and maltodextrin
- Glucose syrup
- Corn syrup and high-fructose corn syrup
- Saccharin
- Aspartame

Variations of the Paleo Diet

One of the best aspects of the Paleo diet is that it can be customized to your specific health needs or conditions as well as dietary requirements, such as food allergies, religious protocols, or conscientious restrictions.

Autoimmune Paleo

The autoimmune protocol (also known as AIP) is a branch of the Paleo diet that eliminates certain foods that are associated with inflammatory responses, particularly in people with chronic and autoimmune disorders like fibromyalgia, eczema, rheumatoid arthritis, lupus, multiple sclerosis, IBS, and Crohn's disease. Nightshades are avoided (including potatoes, tomatoes, and peppers), along with most nuts and seeds and eggs. This food plan is appropriate for individuals who know they're sensitive to any of those foods and for others who are starting Paleo in a compromised state of health.

The Primal Diet

The Primal diet is similar to the Paleo diet with the exception that Primal eating allows organic and raw dairy products, along with fermented soy products and some legumes. Other than that, they follow the same principles of whole foods that are as unprocessed and locally sourced as possible.

While butter isn't a Paleo food (it's Primal), it contains such a low amount of lactose (the sugar found in dairy products that is often difficult to digest) that many Paleo eaters include small amounts of grass-fed, organic butter in their Paleo diets, particularly when mixed with coffee to make what is known as Bulletproof Coffee, a beverage created by author Dave Asprey.

Ketogenic Paleo

The ultimate in low-carb, a ketogenic diet aims to get the body into a state of ketosis where fat is the primary fuel instead of glucose. Ketogenic eating can be 100 percent Paleo compliant and is primarily used by people who have large amounts of weight to lose, as well as bodybuilders, diabetics, and people with other chronic conditions that don't respond well to higher-carb diets.

Pegan

Pegan is short for "Paleo Vegan" and is exactly what it sounds like: a Paleo diet that excludes all animal-based foods. While standard Paleo principles are based on the nourishing benefits of animal products that have been ethically raised and sourced, this version of Paleo focuses strongly on plant-based protein, fats, and produce, and is primarily for those who feel principally or religiously opposed to eating animals.

Food Allergies

Even if you have specific food allergies or sensitivities, the Paleo diet can be fully adapted to work for your dietary requirements without sacrificing quality or convenience. Paleo naturally excludes common allergenic foods such as gluten, corn, soy, peanuts, and artificial sweeteners and additives, but can be adapted for those who are also allergic to eggs, coconut, tree nuts, shellfish, and more.

How do I know what version of the Paleo diet I should follow?
If you're just starting out on the Paleo diet, start by following the basic Paleo food plan. This will give you time to adapt to the new way of eating and evaluate how it impacts your overall health. If you don't see the health improvement you desire, consider implementing one of the stricter versions of Paleo, such as the AIP.

Why Paleo Works

Paleo works as a diet because of its whole-body, health-supportive approach. Regardless of what your wellness goals are, Paleo can help you reach them because it is anti-inflammatory, nourishing, and enables your digestive system to work without hindrance. Without a digestive system that can effectively absorb nutrients, you will never be able to experience true health.

Paleo also works because you can fully make it your Paleo diet. Humans are all uniquely different from one another, and no "one size fits all" approach could ever be truly effective or impactful. Paleo takes the ancient principles of the hunter-gatherer diet and combines them with the knowledge of modern nutrition science, making it a long-lasting, sustainable way of living. Once you've reached your health, fitness, or weight-loss goal, you can continue eating a Paleo diet without still "dieting." The Paleo diet is more of a long-term, wellness-based food plan than it is an actual "diet," which is what makes it so effective for healing Hashimoto's and other chronic and autoimmune disorders.

Are Supplements, Vitamins, Herbs, and Homeopathy Paleo?

If you're switching to a Paleo, whole-food diet, one of the most common questions is do you need to supplement with anything, and if you do, what are the Paleo options? The answer to that question depends on your answers to the following:

- Do you have any chronic or autoimmune disorders?
- Do you have any digestive, intestinal, or malabsorption issues?
- Do you have hormonal imbalances, including thyroid disorders or disease?
- Are you over the age of 60?
- Are you pregnant, trying to become pregnant, or lactating?
- Are you prone to frequent colds, flus, and other viral infections?
- Do you have more than 40 pounds to lose?
- Do you suffer from inflammatory, arthritic, or pain disorders?

If you answered "yes" to any of the previous questions, then it's likely that you could benefit from some form of supplementation. But what and how much? The following guidelines will help you determine what might be beneficial.

ALERT

Just because a product is marketed as "organic" or "natural" doesn't mean that it's compliant with a Paleo diet. The FDA doesn't regulate usage of the word *natural*, so companies can claim that about virtually any product. *Organic* is a term that is more closely regulated, especially when it's USDA certified, but not all organic products will meet Paleo requirements.

Vitamins

Every existing vitamin can be found in supplemental form, in single, combination, and multivitamin formulas. Because food isn't as nutrient-dense as it was back in the Paleolithic era, almost every human can benefit from taking a daily multiple supplement containing the basic vitamins and minerals. From there, people with chronic conditions, like Hashimoto's, can benefit from taking some additional nutrients. Keep in mind that the quality and contents of supplements can vary widely from one brand to another, so it's essential to consult a qualified practitioner for advice and recommendations when choosing vitamin supplements.

In general, supplements from big-box stores are not as high quality as professional brands available from health food stores and practitioners, and many have even been found to contain unlisted fillers such as gluten, soy, and corn. Even some health food store brands and professional brands can contain fillers or other ingredients that aren't Paleo, so you'll want to read the supplement facts on the bottle label carefully. Avoid ingredients that are clearly identifiable as non-Paleo foods (such as wheat, corn, soy, and rice) and anything that is hard to pronounce or not easily recognizable as food.

Herbs

The herbal supplement market is vast, which can easily lead to confusion. You can find herbs marketed for just about every symptom and condition under the sun, but because the FDA doesn't regulate herbal supplements, you need to take all claims with a grain of salt. If herbal products sound too good to be true, they almost certainly are. Additionally, herbs can be quite potent and can cause physical harm if they're not taken according to recommendations, or if they're taken in combination with certain other herbs or medications. This is why it's always a good idea to get your herbs vetted by a nutrition or medical professional who is well versed in herbalism and who can make appropriate recommendations.

It's also important to bear in mind that supplements will never be able to fix or undo a poor diet. They should simply be used to "supplement" or complement a healthy eating plan. When you consider adding herbal support to your Paleo diet, you should be looking to boost specific areas of weakness, not to fix your whole problem or condition.

Homeopathy

Homeopathic products, unlike herbs and vitamins, are regulated by the FDA, and labels on homeopathic products will read as "drug facts." The benefit of homeopathic products is that since they're much more rigidly regulated than other forms of supplements there is less risk for "overdose" or doing potential harm to your body. They are also widely available in health food stores, but as with all dietary supplements, it's a good idea to get professional advice on product choice and dosage.

71

Choosing Quality Supplements

When you're in the market for dietary supplements, here are some key points to keep in mind:

- **Read the complete label, including active and inactive ingredients.** Avoid ingredients that are clearly not Paleo or are hard to pronounce, as these are often not whole-food based.
- **Choose quality brands.** While you don't necessarily need to buy the most expensive option, usually the cheapest one will provide you with the cheapest quality, too. Avoid products from big-box stores and stick to whole-food-based brands that are certified organic. A qualified practitioner can provide you with trusted recommendations.
- **Avoid megadosing unless specifically recommend by a practitioner.** When you supplement single nutrients in large doses you can displace absorption of other nutrients, creating further imbalance within the body. While it's often okay to exceed recommended daily amounts (RDA) of nutrients, since those are set at a base level to avoid deficiency and not to achieve optimal wellness, you don't want to take inordinate amounts of nutrients without proper professional supervision.
- **Pay special attention to fat-soluble nutrients, which can reach toxic levels within the body.** These include fat-soluble vitamins such as vitamins A, D, E, and K, as well as omega fatty acids. With the exception of vitamin D, fat-soluble nutrient needs can be met in your diet by eating a Paleo diet and moderately supplementing with single, daily servings of a multivitamin and fish oil. Vitamin D falls under a special category since it can be produced within the body in response to skin exposure to direct sun rays. Because vitamin D, although not often, can reach toxic levels, it's essential to have your vitamin D levels tested before supplementing with greater than 5,000 IU daily. In cases of low vitamin D, supplementation of 10,000 IU or greater can be helpful for a short duration, but should only be attempted when directed by a professional who will continue to monitor levels. Optimizing vitamin D levels is an essential part of managing and healing Hashimoto's thyroiditis.

ALERT

Essential oils often fall under the category of supplements, but caution should be used with them. Because they're unregulated and highly concentrated substances, use of essential oils should be restricted to those applied topically (when properly mixed with carrier oils) or ones diffused in the air. Essential oils should never be taken internally.

Special Dietary Notes for Hashimoto's

If you have Hashimoto's thyroiditis, which is an autoimmune condition, does that mean that you need to eat the AIP diet? Not necessarily.

The Paleo diet, as a whole, is an anti-inflammatory food plan that promotes digestive wellness and balance within the body. As such, it's a great healing protocol for Hashimoto's disease. Some people who have additional autoimmune disorders or who have been sick for a very long time may need to be stricter on their Paleo diet by following the AIP for a short time. Others who have specific food sensitivities or allergies, particularly to eggs or nuts, will thrive best if they follow the AIP long term.

Even if you don't plan to stick to a Paleo diet forever, certain foods, when broken down in the digestive system, can actually resemble thyroid tissue. If you suffer from leaky gut and these food particles enter your bloodstream, your immune system can become activated and create antibodies against those foods, which translate into antibodies created against your thyroid. These foods that can spark an autoimmune reaction against specific body organs are known as cross-reactive foods, and should be avoided at all times. Gluten and dairy products have cross-reactive properties with the thyroid, so even if you don't follow a strict Paleo diet forever, you should always be mindful to avoid these specific foods that can worsen or destabilize your autoimmune disease.

How to Succeed When Transitioning to a Paleo Diet

Making a major dietary shift can feel overwhelming, but it doesn't have to be! Here are some steps you can take to ensure a successful switch to a Paleo diet.

Understand Your Personality

Some people do best when they make "cold turkey" switches and get rid of all non-Paleo foods in one fell swoop. To make this kind of dietary switch effective, take a day to completely rid your kitchen of all noncompliant foods so they won't be there to confuse or tempt you. Hit the store for a shopping trip prior to your first day of Paleo so that you have what you need to get you through those first few days without the added frustration of trying to go shopping or figure out what you can eat.

Others will be set up for success when they make a gradual transition to a new dietary plan, and this can happen in one of two ways. The first way involves only buying new food that fits the Paleo guidelines, but continuing to eat whatever non-Paleo food is already in your kitchen or pantry. This allows for a more subtle shift over the course of a few days or a few weeks and happens naturally by process of elimination. The other gradual way to switch is to eliminate one non-Paleo category at a time, first going dairy-free, then gluten-free, then grain-free, and so on. This transition takes the longest, but can also feel the most like a solid lifestyle change.

Set Up a Support System

Making a dietary change is a big deal, and even if you're doing it for all the right reasons and you're excited, you will want to have a support system in place so that when you're struggling or having a weak moment, you're not alone. This can come in the form of family members or friends who are going to eat Paleo with you, or by seeking out the counsel of a professional nutritionist or health coach who can keep you accountable and give you motivational tips when you need them.

Don't Aim for Perfection

Being a Paleo perfectionist might seem like it's the fastest way to get healthy, but it can also set you up for a stressful experience. Yes, it's important in the healing process of Hashimoto's to eliminate all non-Paleo foods, but it's also important to manage your stress levels, so don't lose your mind over following the rules. Because it's a lifestyle change and not a temporary diet program, you have time to learn the plan, and after a while, it will become second nature. You won't always have to consult your shopping list of Paleo do's and don'ts and you won't always need to reference recipes when you're trying to cook Paleo meals, but give yourself time to adjust and adapt. Allow for extra time at the supermarket, because reading labels takes time. Learning the products and brands that are Paleo-compliant takes time. Figuring out the recipes you like takes time. There will be slip-ups and cravings, and while you'll want to get back on the Paleo train after they happen, it's certainly not the end of the world when they do.

Plan and Prep

One of the most effective ways to make Paleo a successful and easy lifestyle is to plan ahead. This often includes choosing the meals you intend to make ahead of time, shopping for a week's worth of food at a time, and then taking a few hours or a day to prepare all of your fresh ingredients. This can include washing and cutting vegetables, premeasuring dry ingredients for baked goods, and even batch cooking ahead of time and freezing single-serving or family-sized meal portions.

ESSENTIAL

One creative way to prep vegetables ahead of time is to use a spiralizer to cut them into noodles or thin strips and then freeze for later use. Spiralized vegetables are versatile and can be used in paleoized versions of traditional favorites like spaghetti or chicken noodle soup.

There is no right or wrong way to go about optimizing Paleo to fit your lifestyle, but it will go a long way toward aiding in your success if you plan and prep in ways that make sense for both your personality and your preferences.

How to Eat Your Way to Health

The process of switching to a Paleo diet and focusing on healing your Hashimoto's is not one that will happen overnight. It is a health journey. While many people respond rapidly to the lifestyle changes that come with Paleo eating, you should keep in mind that the average expectation for healing is twice as long as you've been experiencing negative symptoms. While many problematic issues will be resolved quite fast, such as heartburn and bloating, it can take a long time to perceive any changes with others (like inflammation, energy levels, hormone balance, and insomnia). Weight loss sometimes happens rapidly, but since the thyroid is such a sensitive organ, and it regulates metabolism, sometimes it can take weeks or even months to lose weight after changing to a Paleo diet.

The biggest mistake that new Paleo eaters can make is expecting fast results and giving up when they don't happen. Especially when autoimmune disease is present, it's important to take a long-term view. In order to maintain motivation, it can be helpful to keep a record of progress during and after the switch to Paleo eating. This can come in the form of a food journal, progress pictures, weekly weigh-ins, measurements, or mood tracking. Regularly evaluate the areas that are your biggest health complaints and note any progress, as well as improving and/or worsening symptoms. This can serve to keep you on track, with your eyes on the prize, when it feels like nothing is changing.

CHAPTER 5

Adopting the Paleo Lifestyle

Much more than a simple diet, Paleo embodies principles that extend to every aspect of life. If you're going to make the effort to clean up your eating—especially when you're trying to recover from an autoimmune disorder and a compromised state of health—it makes little or no sense not to also take a detailed look at other sources of toxins in your life. Reducing sources of pollutants and chemicals is a great way to help reduce your systemic inflammatory load, not to mention preventively look out for your total body wellness.

Protecting Yourself from Toxins

Toxins are everywhere. You breathe them, eat them, smell them, touch them, and absorb them. The human body is amazingly designed to be able to collect and expel toxins and chemicals, but the volume of pollutants that exist today is dramatically higher than was present several hundred years ago. Even in the last two decades alone, the chances of encountering toxins have dramatically risen, and it is not coincidental that chronic, autoimmune, and inflammatory disorders have also substantially increased.

While there is little you can do to avoid total exposure to all toxins, there are certainly numerous steps you can take to reduce your body's chemical burden and promote clean living not only in your body, but also in your personal space.

QUESTION

What does it mean to "paleoize"? Is that even a real word?
If you search for the word *paleoize* in a dictionary, you will probably come up short. But it is a word that is used within the Paleo community and it refers to the process of swapping non-Paleo or toxic products for Paleo-friendly and clean products. This is applicable to dietary choices as well as body care, home environment, and even mental wellness.

Paleoize Your Home

As you go through the process of paleoizing your diet, you will undoubtedly clean up the contents of your refrigerator, your pantry cabinet, and yes—your gut. These new clean swaps can have revolutionary effects on your physical health, but why stop there? Cleaning products can be a major source of chemicals and contamination. The Environmental Working Group and other environmental experts say that the average American household contains more than sixty chemicals, but it need not stay that way. You live in the age of DIY and going back to the way your ancestors did it before all the products of modern "convenience" existed. The Paleo community has thoroughly embraced the cleaning power of natural ingredients such as baking soda, vinegar, lemon, borax, and essential oils, among other nontoxic things. It is entirely possible to throw away your bleach and never look back. Plus, most of these natural ingredients don't pose a risk to you, your child, or your pet. That is definitely not the case with most conventional cleaning products.

Here's a summary of several of the most common toxic household chemicals:

- **Diethylene glycol:** This common solvent found in glass cleaners is poisonous if ingested (although, which items on this list aren't?), and suppresses nervous system function.
- **1,4-Dioxane:** This solvent is used in laundry detergents, even some "free and clear" detergents, and has been associated with an increased risk in breast cancer, according to a report by Women's Voices for the Earth.
- **Perchloroethylene:** This neurotoxin is found in carpet cleaners, upholstery spot cleaners, and even in dry-cleaning solutions (home or professional). Avoid these products or find nontoxic alternatives (such as steam cleaning instead of dry cleaning).
- **Ammonia:** One of the more well known (and pronounceable) ingredients, ammonia is a strong skin irritant. It is found in many window and glass cleaning products, as well as those aimed at the kitchen and bathroom.
- **Phthalates:** Generally found in anything with scent or fragrance, these are endocrine disruptors that have a dramatic impact on men and women. But don't expect to always see these on labels since companies don't have to disclose every ingredient that comprises their trademarked "fragrance." If you see the word *fragrance* or if the product is scented, chances are that the product contains these chemicals.
- **Chlorine:** Found in most sources of city tap water, chlorine exposure can quickly multiply based on water exposure and presence in cleaning products like toilet and sink scrubbers, bleach alternatives, and mold/mildew cleaners. This is of special concern for patients with Hashimoto's, as the thyroid is particularly sensitive to chlorine exposure, so it's essential to eliminate chlorinated products and to filter water if it is chlorinated.
- **Galaxolide:** A synthetic fragrance often found in air-purifying products, this is a hormone disruptor that should be avoided by all Hashimoto's patients.

- **Corrosive chemicals:** This is a general category of household cleaners that include oven and stovetop cleaner, drain cleaners and decloggers, and foaming toilet bowl scrub. These cleaners come with warnings on the product labels indicating that skin irritation, burns, or lung damage can occur if they touch the skin or if their fumes are breathed in. They can also irritate or burn the eyes as a result of the gases that they give off during the "cleaning" process.
- **Triclosan:** This chemical has received a lot of publicity in recent years. As the microbiome is researched more, this chemical, which is part of antibacterial products, is found to be incredibly harmful to the beneficial bacteria in the human gut. It can also contribute to the development of "superbugs" or antibiotic-resistant bacteria. Humans thrive in nonsterile environments, so plain, fragrance-free soap is more than sufficient for cleaning away germs. In fact, humans require the presence of many different forms of nonharmful bacteria to thrive, and triclosan damages those, too.

FACT

Companies that manufacture cleaning products, body care products, or cosmetics are not required to disclose every ingredient contained within. This means that a number of toxic chemical ingredients may not be listed on any given product label, and "free and clear" or "natural" products are not excepted! The only way to completely eliminate all chemicals from your home is to make your own cleaning products or to purchase from companies that voluntarily disclose all their ingredients.

Instead of using chemicals to "clean" your house by swapping dirt for damaging toxins (when did society get so dirt and germ phobic, anyway?), the following items can be used to make your own household cleaners that are equally or more effective. There is a plethora of cleaning resources online, and some are listed in Appendix B if you would like to further explore this.

- White vinegar
- Baking soda
- Lemon juice
- Borax

- Water
- Castile soap
- Sponge
- Microfiber cloth
- Olive oil
- Coconut oil
- Essential oils, especially tea tree oil, eucalyptus, lemon, lavender, and peppermint
- Vodka
- Washing soda

Paleoize Your Medicine Cabinet

Perhaps *medicine cabinet* is a vague term, but when it comes to daily body care and first aid, the drugstore industry has this market cornered. Still, the volume of toxins that we take in from anything like toothpaste to shampoo to hair spray to body lotion is staggering. There are natural alternatives to everything, and whether you make them or buy them, you're investing in the long-term future of your body. By spending a little more money on things in the present, you are literally bettering your future. Toxic and chemical-laden body care products may not seem that damaging in the short term, but that is where they get you: The cumulative impact of using them day in and day out for years and even decades is what causes the slow descent into toxicity, cellular degeneration, inflammation, and even cancer.

FACT

While the FDA regulates prescription drugs and homeopathic products, it does not regulate supplements. Body care items and cosmetics are not regulated, either. While the general assumption is that companies can't sell products known to be damaging or toxic, this is simply not true. Instead of granting companies (which are profiting from your purchases) the benefit of doubt, start doing your research and make them prove to you why their products should be purchased. Simply reading the labels on most drugstore beauty products will be enough to make you question the use of so many chemicals.

Following is a list of common toxins found in body care and first-aid products. For more information on chemical-free replacements, consult the Environmental Working Group's online database at www.ewg.org/skindeep.

- **DEA, TEA, and MEA:** Foaming agents in shampoo, body wash, bubble bath, soap
- **Formaldehyde:** Preservative used in hair dye, nail polish, shampoo, body wash
- **Parfum:** Another way of saying "synthetic fragrance"
- **Mercury:** Preservative found in mascara
- **Petroleum and mineral oil:** Moisturizers found in lotions, diaper rash cream, hair gel
- **Sodium lauryl sulfate:** Soap foamer used in body wash, shampoo
- **Talc:** Powdery substance used to make eye shadow, blush, foundation, powder
- **FD&C:** Pigmentation ingredients derived from coal tar

Paleoize Your Cosmetics

It's possible to have the cleanest diet, the greenest house, and the most organic body care regimen and to still be slathering on dozens of chemicals on a daily basis in the form of cosmetics, perfumes, and nail polish. These items are separated here from body care items because these tend to apply (for the most part) to female grooming routines, and therefore, increase a woman's exposure to toxicity much more significantly than a man's. Is it coincidental, then, that women experience Hashimoto's eight times more than men? While this is largely due to the greater volume of hormones that women have, when hormones go awry because of environmental factors, the consequences are more severe.

So what's in lipstick or mascara? As a matter of fact, all forms of drug-store makeup, and even some more natural brands, contain chemicals, hormone disruptors, and toxins that are stacking up to cause quite a burden on your body, particularly your liver and your endocrine organs. The liver is responsible for getting toxins out of your body once they've gotten in, and your endocrine organs become confused with all the extra noise that comes from hormone disruptors. With Hashimoto's disease, the thyroid is going to be even more susceptible to inflammation from these outside sources, making it vital for you to really understand what is going on your face. Can you really justify pampering yourself when it is adding to the inflammatory load of your body?

ALERT

The average age at which girls first experience menstruation is getting younger and younger, largely due to the widespread presence of endocrine disruptors. These hormone-signaling ingredients get into the body and send messages to the endocrine organs, including the thyroid, adrenal glands, and reproductive organs. These endocrine disruptors are found in foods, household products, body care items, and especially cosmetics. It is essential to carefully monitor the chemical burden that preteen and teenage girls encounter to avoid potential long-term consequences.

The great news is that along with all the other categories, organic and chemical-free makeup is increasing in popularity and is much more widely available, along with perfumes, nail polish, and the like. You can still pamper yourself and feel beautiful, and as a bonus, you can feel confident in the fact that you're furthering your wellness journey, not hindering it.

Here is a sampling of ingredients frequently found in drugstore cosmetics:

- **Parabens:** These can be listed on the label as methylparaben, propylparaben, or ethylparaben. They're used primarily as preservatives.
- **BHT:** Butylated hydroxytoluene, toluene, benzoic, or benzyl; these are fat-soluble preservatives used to retain product coloring. They aren't limited to cosmetics, however; they are also found in embalming fluid. If that doesn't make you put the product back on the shelf, maybe nothing will.
- **DMDM hydantoin:** Another form of preservative, but this one releases toxic formaldehyde into the body.
- **Phthalates:** These have plastic-like qualities that give makeup a spongier or thicker texture, and are also found in nail polishes and perfume. They can be listed on labels as DEP, DBP, DEHP, or others. These chemicals specifically have been identified not only as cancer-causing, but they are also major endocrine disruptors for girls and boys, resulting in early

onset puberty and estrogen dominance in girls and testosterone reduction in boys.

- **Fragrance:** Many cosmetics beyond just perfume have fragrance added, but most fragrances are just synthetic chemical cocktails. Fragrance chemicals can include ethanol, acetone, and methylene chloride, among several others. You don't have to understand chemical jargon on a label to avoid this category of chemicals: If it has a scent that isn't clearly demonstrated to be from real, earthborn scents (like essential oils, plants, or flowers), avoid it. Fragrance-free is the way to be.

ALERT

Beth Greer's book *Super Natural Home* discusses a study done by Shanna Swan, PhD, in 2006. The study examined how phthalates impacted development of boys *in utero* and after they were born. Boys exposed to the most phthalates from their pregnant mothers were more likely to have smaller penises and/or undescended testicles. That is some serious endocrine disruption right there, with lifelong consequences. For more information on the total lifestyle consequences of toxins, and for a way into cleaner personal living, check out her book.

Instead of choosing synthetic makeup, consider the following ingredients that natural, chemical-free makeups utilize. You can purchase quality products, or you can even make your own!

- Activated charcoal
- Almond oil
- Aloe vera
- Argan oil
- Arrowroot powder
- Avocado oil
- Beeswax
- Calendula
- Clay
- Cocoa butter
- Cocoa powder

- Coconut milk
- Coconut oil
- Essential oils
- Gelatin
- Jojoba oil
- Kukui oil
- Lanolin
- Lavender
- Olive oil
- Rose water
- Shea butter
- Spirulina
- Vegetable glycerin
- Vitamin E oil
- Zinc oxide

Any number of food, herbal, or flower ingredients can be used to naturally color your homemade makeup. For more information on making your own cosmetic products, consult Appendix B.

Paleoize Your Thinking—Mind-Body Health and Autoimmunity

Not only are mood disorders a common side effect of thyroid disease, they're also strongly associated with autoimmune reactivity in general. According to the research presented in the textbook *Mind Body Health: The Effects of Attitudes, Emotions, and Relationships*, authors Keith J. Karren, N. Lee Smith, and Kathryn J. Gordon explain that every part of the immune system is connected to the brain in one way or another. The brain by way of the nervous system communicates extensively with the immune system. Lymphocytes, which are a specific type of white blood cell, contain receptacles on their surfaces for messages to and from the nervous system. The messages being sent involve hormones, including those of the thyroid. These receptors on the lymphocytes enable channels of communication in both directions between the nervous system and the immune system, but it also means that the immune system is capable of receiving messages of both physical and psychological stress.

Stress causes the brain to release neurohormones that can bind with lymphocytes, and that can literally alter immune function and capability. But the brain and the immune system are linked in other ways, too. Peptides are chemical messengers that were once thought to be produced only by the brain and endocrine organs, but they're also produced in the immune system. Peptides transmit information throughout the body about not only physical function, but emotional function as well. Again, according to Karren, Smith, and Gordon, this could explain the link between negative emotions, stress, and reduced immunity or autoimmunity. When the immune system receives peptides carrying negative emotions or overwhelming amounts of stress, and these continue for some time, the body becomes exhausted from producing physical responses to it. Reduced immunity, greater susceptibility to sickness, and autoimmune reactions can result.

Stress, Mindfulness, and Hashimoto's

So can negative emotions or stress cause Hashimoto's thyroiditis? As much as some natural health authors would have people believe that all disease is rooted in negative emotions, and that people can easily heal themselves if they change their thinking, that is a very limiting view and fails to take into account genetic individuality, environmental factors, endocrine disruptors, and the cascade effect of multiple autoimmune disorders. What is most likely the case is that once a condition is present, negative emotions can certainly further weaken the body or perpetuate existing physical conditions. But does one single negative thought become another and another and spark disease in a perfectly healthy individual? And on the flip side, can positive thinking and a state of emotional contentment and well-being actually heal the body, without any other factors?

The impact of mind-body health cannot be discounted in a healing plan, and certainly human ancestors from the hunter-gatherer days did not have the influx of negative emotions and stress that plague modern society. But focusing on mindfulness alone, without also introducing a restorative eating plan, balancing hormones, and reducing chemical exposure and toxicity, will not be successful for entering remission with Hashimoto's disease.

Paleoize Your Fitness

Paleo and CrossFit have become synonymous in some circles, but do you have to do CrossFit if you enter a Paleo lifestyle? No, you don't, and in fact, there's a good chance that you shouldn't. Paleo is about intuitively eating and altering your lifestyle to equip your body to function at its best. This will mean different things for different people, but when you have an autoimmune disease, and a hormone-based one at that, there are many downsides to intense exercise like that of CrossFit. Distance running, weightlifting, and other forms of fitness that raise your heart rate to maximum levels will actually deplete the body of T3, causing longer recovery times, exercise intolerance, and adrenal fatigue.

ESSENTIAL

Another exercise program that is health restorative is known as T-Tapp, named after creator Teresa Tapp. While it may initially feel quirky, the value in the workout is that it's low impact and short (just 15 minutes). Many people who follow the program report effects of lowered blood glucose and cholesterol, as well as increased hormone balance. You can find more information about the program at www.t-tapp.com.

Adopting a healing lifestyle for Hashimoto's isn't about pushing yourself to the max. It's about slowing down and listening to your body. Many patients who end up being diagnosed with thyroid disease will recognize that feeling of being rundown, perhaps for months or even years. When you're feeling that kind of burnout, along with other symptoms of Hashimoto's, you don't want to pile stress onto your body as it is trying to heal. Even though exercise is "good for you," it can be too much in this restorative phase.

So while you shouldn't knock yourself out to become a marathon runner or a CrossFit Games champion, you definitely should get regular with a calmer form of exercise. Programs like yoga, Pilates, and barre workouts are excellent for health restoration because they address stress levels while also working muscles and burning moderate amounts of calories. Even though you may have thyroid-induced weight to lose, killing yourself through intense workout routines is not the way to go about it. Doing this might produce some short-term weight loss, but long-term, you will most likely experience an extreme rise in fatigue, constantly fluctuating thyroid hormone levels, and ultimately, a spike in your overall autoimmunity.

Does this mean that you can never be a runner or a weightlifting athlete? No, but you need to take a long view of your healing process. It does most likely mean that for a good couple of years you need to focus on energy-boosting, healing, and therapeutic ways to move your body: Walking, light swimming, yoga, Pilates, tai chi, and barre are going to produce the best results, especially when practiced regularly over time.

Creating a Successful Self-Care Plan

You now have the tools needed to create and implement a self-care plan to address your Hashimoto's, as well as any other existing autoimmune or chronic conditions. Here are ten points to consider as you move forward in your journey toward healing and antibody remission:

1. **Your age:** While you can enter a healing path for Hashimoto's at any age, keep in mind that your age may play a significant role in how quickly your body responds to treatment and lifestyle adjustments. The length of time you have been sick will also be an important factor to consider. Has your Hashimoto's been undiagnosed for years or even a decade or longer? You will likely take more time to enter remission than someone who discovered her thyroid antibodies before she was clinically hypothyroid.

2. **Your current level of antibodies:** If your antibodies are only slightly elevated, you will likely be in remission shortly after beginning a health-supportive program. If they are sky-high, on the other hand, coming in at hundreds or thousands, you have to accept that it will take time for your body to cool from that level of inflammation. It takes time for the immune system to receive the message that it can calm down, and it takes time for the thyroid to respond to the cessation of auto-antibody attacks.

3. **Your current weight:** If you only have 5–10 pounds to lose, this may happen rather quickly as inflammation subsides, but it is not uncommon for Hashimoto's patients with 20 or more pounds to lose to feel like it takes a significant amount of time before they see the weight budge. This can be due to a slow implementation of a Hashimoto's healing program (e.g.,

easing into a Paleo diet, and continuing to eat foods that are cross-reactive for some length of time), or a result of another undiagnosed autoimmune disorder, or simply your personal reaction to adjusting to a new health pattern. The body doesn't actually do change well. It prefers to keep things stable and balanced, and if you've been sick for a long time, even though it's not optimal, it is familiar. It's all right if it takes some time. There are far more determinant factors for health than the number on the scale.

4. **Your current level of fitness:** Are you a recovering fitness addict who enjoyed training for marathons or running miles a day? You may find this new "restorative exercise" program to be frustrating. As a result, you may have trouble fully giving up your intense workouts and may slow down your path to wellness. This isn't necessarily bad; it's just a fact to be considered in your approach to healing. Are you a fitness beginner? Have you been too tired to exercise for years? Start slow. Don't begin an exercise program, even one that involves yoga or walking, and expect to be working out 5–7 days a week. Your body will still need to adjust to new levels of movement, so begin by trying short workouts 3 days a week. They can be 5 minutes or 15 minutes. At this point it isn't the length of time that matters so much as getting into the pattern of healing movement.

5. **Your job:** Is your job highly stressful? Do you work long hours or travel often? You will need to factor these details into your healing plan. A person who works from home or has a predictable, low-stress job will respond faster to lifestyle adjustments because there will be fewer physical stressors. People with higher-stress jobs or more fast-paced lifestyles can certainly still implement a healing program, but it will need to be more intentionally carved out and adhered to.

6. **Your food preferences:** Paleo is adaptable for your food preferences, tastes, and desired level of dietary elimination. The recipes in this book are all Paleo, and a good portion of them are also AIP friendly. Some of them are Pegan, and others may fall within the nutrient ranges for a ketogenic diet. Ideally, you will eat through a variety of these Paleo recipes, perhaps alternating between the sample food plans. This will introduce you to a wide range of nutrients from foods, which is the best way to

receive them and absorb them. If specific foods are problematic, many easy food swaps can be made to customize the plan for you.

7. **Your finances:** Paleo can be as expensive as you want it to be. Even the existing meal plans in this book can be adapted for any budget. Swap out more widely available and less-expensive vegetables for the less-common ones; buy fruit in bulk and freeze it; buy meat in bulk directly from butchers. The Internet is rife with cheap ways to eat Paleo, and Appendix B contains some resources to get you started on your journey.

8. **Your support network:** You can be a one-man or one-woman show quite easily when switching to a Paleo lifestyle, but any major change or health commitment will be easier when you have one or more persons in your life who are cheering you on. Whether it is a partner, a parent, a sibling, a child, a friend, or a coworker, you'll set yourself up for the best chance of success if you have someone to turn to when the going gets rough or when you're super tempted by non-Paleo food. If there isn't anyone in your life who can support you, there are numerous online communities devoted to the Paleo lifestyle, as well as others focusing on thyroid disease and autoimmunity in general.

9. **Your goals:** While you may share goals with many others who have thyroid disease, they will naturally differ in some ways due to the unique factors that make up your life. Goals can range from physical (lose weight, get healthy), to mental (have more energy, beat depression), to emotional (feel better about yourself, feel a sense of accomplishment), but are often a combination of all the above. It's good to set both short-term and long-term goals. Short-term goals will keep you motivated as you constantly experience the success of completing them, much like climbing a ladder. Long-term goals will take more time and concerted effort to achieve, but the short-term goals should all be leading to the end game of greater wellness and, hopefully, remission and healing from Hashimoto's.

10. **Your willingness:** Ultimately, no one is in charge of your success except for you. Doctors and other health practitioners will be there to support you along the way, but you're the only person who can feel and sense exactly what is happening within your body and your cells. Cultivate that sense of intuition and personal connectedness, and use it to develop a dogged insistence that you will not quit until you are where you want to be.

QUESTION

Where can I find online support for a Paleo lifestyle?
Numerous Paleo websites have blogs written by experts, offer nutritionist-guided community challenges, moderate interactive forums, and utilize social media to connect with followers. Some of the more popular Paleo websites that offer support, especially for those new to the Paleo lifestyle, include Paleo Plan (www.paleoplan.com), Paleo Leap (http://paleoleap.com), and Paleo Grubs (http://paleogrubs.com).

When Will You Feel "Normal" Again?

The concept of normality is one that probably shouldn't be mentioned in the context of health or wellness. What is normal, anyway?

When most people ask this question, they are wondering when they will feel as good or better than they used to, and that is a valid question. The answer is different for everyone. Most people who thoroughly implement lifestyle and dietary changes to address Hashimoto's will notice some level of improvement within 1–3 months. "Some level of improvement" means that you will notice some positive changes. Your antibodies may decrease, your free T3 and free T4 may stabilize, other labs like cholesterol or glucose may improve, and your digestive health may be noticeably different. But for there to be a total transformation—or a return to the healthful days of your youth or before Hashimoto's came into play—you need to realistically expect for it to take several months to a year, and potentially beyond. It will be a lifelong process of supporting your body, but you should continually feel and see measurable progress. Setting realistic expectations is best done with the help of professionals who can fully assess your individual situation, but if you are content to take things one step at a time, and celebrate each victory as it comes, you will begin to feel better on a number of levels. Healing autoimmunity is an epic endeavor, but one that is well worth the efforts. There is truly no greater reward than health that is fought for and achieved one courageous, persistent step after another.

CHAPTER 6

Fermented Foods, Soups, and Broths

Easy DIY Sauerkraut

Making your own 'kraut at home gives you the benefit of having a preservative-free version that is pure probiotic power for your gut. This version is sweet and tangy and can be eaten plain or added to a salad for extra flavor.

PREP TIME: 3–5 DAYS
COOK TIME: N/A

INGREDIENTS | SERVES 6

1 medium head green cabbage, finely chopped

2 large carrots, peeled and finely chopped

1 small white onion, peeled and finely chopped

1 small Granny Smith apple, cored and finely chopped

1 clove garlic, peeled and finely chopped

⅛ teaspoon finely ground sea salt

Measure It Out

By using a scale, you'll ensure a proper vegetable-to-salt ratio and your 'kraut will taste perfect. You can find these kitchen scales at any grocery store or from online retailers like Amazon.

1. Using a kitchen scale, weigh a medium mixing bowl. Note the measurement.

2. In the mixing bowl, combine cabbage, carrots, onion, apple, and garlic. Mix thoroughly with clean hands. Weigh the mixture on the kitchen scale and subtract the weight of the bowl.

3. For every pound of mixture, measure out ¼ ounce sea salt. Add this to vegetable mixture and continue mixing with hands for a few minutes until mixture starts to release water. Let sit 4–6 hours, stirring every hour.

4. Add vegetable mixture and liquid to a large glass jar, packing vegetables down as tightly as possible. Use a second jar if necessary.

5. Cover the jar with a piece of muslin fabric or cheesecloth, secure a rubber band around the neck, and refrigerate 3–5 days for the fermentation process to take place. Check daily to ensure that there is enough water in the jar, and if necessary, add water ¼ cup at a time. Keep refrigerated.

Per Serving Calories: 54 | Fat: 0.1g | Protein: 2g | Sodium: 86mg | Fiber: 4g | Carbohydrates: 13g | Sugar: 8g

Coconut Kefir Yogurt

This cultured yogurt is perfect for topping fruity desserts or eating by itself for breakfast. Add your favorite berries or Paleo granola for a hearty snack.

PREP TIME: 1–3 DAYS
COOK TIME: N/A

INGREDIENTS | SERVES 10

2 (13.66-ounce) cans full-fat coconut milk

2 tablespoons probiotic powder

2 tablespoons raw honey

Kinds of Coconut Milk

There are different types of coconut milk available to purchase, and for this recipe you'll want the canned kind often found in the Asian foods section. The refrigerated kind of coconut milk is low-fat, and will not be thick enough for this recipe.

1. In a food processor or blender, blend coconut milk until smooth and creamy.

2. Pour blended coconut milk into a medium glass bowl and stir in probiotic powder. Cover bowl with muslin, cheesecloth, or some other form of breathable fabric and secure with a rubber band. Store in a cool, dark place 1–3 days to allow for culturing. The yogurt should have a bite to it, like unsweetened Greek yogurt.

3. Add honey to yogurt and stir. Keep refrigerated up to 1 week.

Per Serving Calories: 165 | Fat: 15.5g | Protein: 2g | Sodium: 10mg | Fiber: 0g | Carbohydrates: 6g | Sugar: 3g

Sweet Orange Pickled Beets

This gives a new, flavorful twist to Grandma's pickled beets. The addition of citrus and honey makes them sweet and the perfect colorful side for any meal or tangy topping for a salad.

PREP TIME: 12 HOURS
COOK TIME: 3–6 HOURS

INGREDIENTS | SERVES 10

5 large beets, peeled and sliced
2 cups water
1 cup white vinegar
Juice of 4 large oranges, divided
2 teaspoons sea salt
½ cup raw honey

Beet Red

Beets will stain your hands, so it's a good idea to wear gloves while handling them. Additionally, only use glass when storing them; other types of containers will be permanently tinged with a beet-red hue.

1. In a 4-quart slow cooker, combine beets, water, vinegar, half the orange juice, and salt. Cover and cook on low heat 6 hours or on high heat 3 hours. Beets should be soft at the center when fully cooked.

2. Remove from slow cooker and drain, setting aside 2 cups cooking liquid. Let cool 30–60 minutes.

3. In a large mixing bowl, combine cooked beets with remaining orange juice, honey, and cooking liquid. Stir thoroughly. Cover and refrigerate overnight before serving. Store in refrigerator up to 10 days.

Per Serving Calories: 84 | Fat: 0.1g | Protein: 1g | Sodium: 492mg | Fiber: 1g | Carbohydrates: 20g | Sugar: 18.5g

AIP Vegetable Soup

The preroasted vegetables give this soup a richer flavor than the average vegetable soup, and the lard adds a creaminess that most Paleo soups lack.

PREP TIME: 10 MINUTES
COOK TIME: 1 HOUR 40 MINUTES

INGREDIENTS | SERVES 6

3 large carrots, peeled and chopped

1 large parsnip, peeled and chopped

4 cloves garlic, peeled and chopped

1 large beet, peeled and chopped

1 large sweet potato, peeled and chopped

6 tablespoons lard

½ teaspoon sea salt

½ teaspoon ground black pepper

1 teaspoon onion powder

6 cups Chicken Stock (see recipe in this chapter)

1. Preheat oven to 375°F. In a large mixing bowl, combine carrots, parsnips, garlic, beet, and potato with lard, salt, pepper, and onion powder. Mix thoroughly so that the vegetables are coated.

2. Spread vegetable mixture evenly on a baking sheet and bake 35–40 minutes or until vegetables are soft.

3. In a large stew pot, combine roasted vegetables with stock and cook on medium heat 1 hour, and then reduce heat to low until ready to serve.

Per Serving Calories: 229 | Fat: 15g | Protein: 5g | Sodium: 738mg | Fiber: 5g | Carbohydrates: 19g | Sugar: 6.5g

Mediterranean Seafood Soup

This quick and easy soup will give you a taste of the Mediterranean.

PREP TIME: 15 MINUTES
COOK TIME: 25 MINUTES

INGREDIENTS | SERVES 2

2 tablespoons olive oil

½ cup chopped sweet onion

2 cloves garlic, peeled and chopped

½ medium bulb fennel, chopped

½ cup Chicken Stock (see recipe in this chapter)

1 cup clam juice

2 cups chopped tomatoes

6 littleneck clams, scrubbed and rinsed

6 mussels, scrubbed and rinsed

8 raw jumbo shrimp, peeled and deveined

1 teaspoon dried basil, or 5 leaves fresh basil, torn

¼ teaspoon sea salt

¼ teaspoon red pepper flakes

1. Heat oil in a large frying pan over medium heat and add onion, garlic, and fennel. After 10 minutes, stir in stock and clam juice and add tomatoes. Bring to a boil.

2. Drop clams into the boiling liquid. When clams start to open, add mussels. When mussels start to open, add shrimp, basil, salt, and pepper flakes. Serve when shrimp turns pink. Discard any unopened clams or mussels.

Per Serving Calories: 361 | Fat: 14g | Protein: 35g | Sodium: 3,004mg | Fiber: 5g | Carbohydrates: 18g | Sugar: 9g

Littleneck Clams

Littleneck clams are the smallest variety of hard-shell clams and can be found off the northeastern and northwestern coasts of the United States. They have a sweet taste and are delicious in soup, steamed and dipped in melted butter, battered and fried, or baked.

Caveman's Cabbage Soup

Slow-cooking cabbage soup preserves the nutrients in the cabbage and other vegetables, versus other, higher-temperature methods of preparation that tend to destroy many of the nutrients. Add cooked sausage slices to the pot for a well-rounded meal.

PREP TIME: 10 MINUTES
COOK TIME: 8–10 HOURS
INGREDIENTS | SERVES 4

1 small head green cabbage, chopped

2 green onions, sliced

1 large red bell pepper, seeded and chopped

4 large stalks celery, chopped

1 cup baby carrots

4 cups Chicken Stock (see recipe in this chapter)

4 cups water

3 cloves garlic, peeled and minced

¼ teaspoon red pepper flakes

¼ teaspoon dried basil

¼ teaspoon dried oregano

¼ teaspoon dried thyme

¼ teaspoon onion powder

Combine all ingredients in a 6-quart slow cooker. Cover and cook on low 8–10 hours.

Per Serving Calories: 39 | Fat: 1g | Protein: 2g | Sodium: 174mg | Fiber: 2g | Carbohydrates: 5g | Sugar: 3g

Ham and Chard Soup

This Paleo spin on ham and potato soup includes chard for an added vegetable boost while also providing the familiar taste of classic comfort food.

PREP TIME: 10 MINUTES
COOK TIME: 5½–11 HOURS

INGREDIENTS | SERVES 6

7 cups Chicken Stock (see recipe in this chapter)

7 ounces ham, cubed

1 large sweet potato, peeled and cubed

1 medium parsnip, peeled and cubed

1 medium turnip, peeled and cubed

4 large carrots, peeled and chopped

2 medium celery stalks, chopped

2 cloves garlic, peeled and chopped

½ teaspoon dried thyme

½ teaspoon ground black pepper

1 teaspoon sea salt

3 cups torn or coarsely chopped chard

1. In a 6-quart slow cooker, combine all ingredients except chard. Cover and cook on high heat 5 hours or on low heat 10 hours.

2. Stir in chard, cover, and cook an additional 30–60 minutes on high heat.

Per Serving Calories: 199 | Fat: 8g | Protein: 11g | Sodium: 1,368mg | Fiber: 5g | Carbohydrates: 20g | Sugar: 7g

Any Greens Will Do
If you don't have chard, you can easily substitute kale, spinach, or beet greens in this recipe for a similar nutritional profile.

Beef and Kelp Noodle Soup

A Paleo twist on beef and noodle soup, this AIP-friendly soup is free of allergens, and thanks to the kelp noodles, it is rich in calcium and fiber.

PREP TIME: 10 MINUTES
COOK TIME: 5–8 HOURS

INGREDIENTS | SERVES 6

3 tablespoons ghee

2 pounds beef steak, cubed

6 cups Beef Stock (see recipe in this chapter)

2 cups Slow-Cooker Beef Bone Broth (see recipe in this chapter)

1 large onion, peeled and finely chopped

4 cloves garlic, peeled and quartered

1 pound portobello mushrooms, halved

3 large carrots, peeled and chopped

3 tablespoons coconut aminos

1 teaspoon sea salt

1 teaspoon ground black pepper

16 ounces kelp noodles

1. Heat a large skillet on medium-high heat 2 minutes and then add ghee. Brown steak and then remove from heat.

2. In a 6-quart slow cooker, combine steak and all other ingredients except kelp noodles. Cover and cook on low 6 hours or on high 3 hours.

3. Add kelp noodles to slow cooker, cover, and cook on high heat 2 more hours. Serve warm.

Per Serving   Calories: 480 | Fat: 29g | Protein: 39g | Sodium: 1,906 | Fiber: 4g | Carbohydrates: 16g | Sugar: 6g

Chicken and Vegetable Garden Soup

*All the comforts of chicken soup with a generous helping of vegetables.
It's a one-dish "soup and salad" wonder!*

PREP TIME: 10 MINUTES
COOK TIME: 4–8 HOURS

INGREDIENTS | SERVES 6

1 large onion, peeled and finely chopped

2 tablespoons ghee

4 cloves garlic, peeled and chopped

4 (8-ounce) boneless, skinless chicken breasts, chopped

10 cups Chicken Stock (see recipe in this chapter)

3 large carrots, peeled and chopped

1 medium head cauliflower, chopped

½ pound portobello mushrooms, halved

2 large parsnips, peeled and chopped

2 large zucchini, chopped

Parsnips, Turnips, and Potatoes

This recipe calls for parsnips because they're AIP-friendly, but you can easily swap parsnips for turnips or white or sweet potatoes, making it a great recipe to use whatever ingredients you have on hand.

1. In a large skillet, combine onion, ghee, garlic, and chicken and cook over medium-high heat 5 minutes or until browned.

2. Add chicken mixture to a 6-quart slow cooker with remaining ingredients. Cover and cook on low heat 8 hours or on high heat 4 hours.

Per Serving Calories: 407 | Fat: 15g | Protein: 42g | Sodium: 875mg | Fiber: 8g | Carbohydrates: 25.5g | Sugar: 10g

Ultra Vegetable Bison Stew

*This recipe swaps beef for bison, and potatoes for turnips,
but even the pickiest of eaters will be satisfied with this classic-tasting stew.*

PREP TIME: 10 MINUTES
COOK TIME: 4–10 HOURS

INGREDIENTS | SERVES 6

1 large onion, peeled and finely chopped

3 tablespoons ghee

4 cloves garlic, peeled and finely chopped

1 cup Chicken Stock (see recipe in this chapter)

1 (6-pound) bison roast

6 cups Beef Stock (see recipe in this chapter)

½ pound portobello mushrooms, halved

¼ cup Worcestershire sauce

2 teaspoons sea salt

1 teaspoon ground black pepper

1 teaspoon garlic powder

1 teaspoon onion powder

2 large sweet potatoes, peeled and chopped

4 large carrots, peeled and chopped

2 large turnips, peeled and chopped

1 large parsnip, peeled and chopped

½ pound kale, torn into ½" pieces

1. In a large skillet over medium-high heat, cook onion in ghee until browned. Add garlic and Chicken Stock and cook until stock begins to boil. Transfer to a 6-quart slow cooker.

2. In the same skillet sear bison over medium-high heat until browned on all sides. Remove and add to slow cooker.

3. Add remaining ingredients to slow cooker, cover, and cook on low heat 8–10 hours or on high heat 4–6 hours.

Per Serving Calories: 853 | Fat: 27.5g | Protein: 106g | Sodium: 2,087mg | Fiber: 8g | Carbohydrates: 38.5g | Sugar: 14g

Thai Chicken Stew

This hearty chicken stew is an exciting blend of ginger, lemon, lime, and honey that invokes the classic "sweet and spicy" flavor profile, while providing a fresh use of these Paleo-friendly ingredients.

PREP TIME: 10 MINUTES
COOK TIME: 6 HOURS 30 MINUTES
INGREDIENTS | SERVES 6

3 pounds boneless, skinless chicken thighs

2 teaspoons sea salt

1 teaspoon ground black pepper

2 cups water

2 large onions, peeled and finely chopped

3 tablespoons ghee

4 cloves garlic, peeled and chopped

2 tablespoons grated fresh ginger

2 cups Chicken Stock (see recipe in this chapter)

4 teaspoons collagen powder

½ cup cold water

1 (13.66-ounce) can full-fat coconut milk

Juice of 2 large limes

Juice of 1 large lemon

1 tablespoon fish sauce

1 tablespoon coconut sugar

½ pound snow peas, stems removed

Fish Sauce

Fish sauce is made from fermented fish stock, and can be found in the Asian cooking aisle at the grocery store. Make sure to read the label for extra ingredients that might not be Paleo-friendly.

1. Add chicken thighs, salt, and pepper to a 6-quart slow cooker with 2 cups water. Turn to high heat and cover.

2. In a large skillet over medium-high heat, sauté onions with ghee, garlic, ginger, and stock about 5 minutes or until onions are browned. Retain liquid in pan and transfer other ingredients to slow cooker.

3. In a small mixing bowl, sprinkle collagen over cold water and let sit 3–5 minutes to soften and absorb water.

4. Combine liquid from skillet and collagen mixture. Whisk rapidly until mixture is fully combined. Add to slow cooker and cook 4 hours on high heat.

5. In a small saucepan over medium heat, combine coconut milk, lime, lemon, fish sauce, and coconut sugar. Stir frequently until thoroughly combined. Once hot, add mixture to slow cooker along with snow peas. Cook an additional 2 hours on high heat.

6. Remove chicken and shred with a fork. Return chicken to soup and serve warm.

Per Serving Calories: 526 | Fat: 28.5g | Protein: 49.5g | Sodium: 1,428mg | Fiber: 3g | Carbohydrates: 15g | Sugar: 7g

Green Pork Chili

This colorful twist on classic chili uses pork instead of red meat and jalapeños instead of red chili powder. You can customize the level of spiciness to your personal palate by using more or less jalapeños. To keep it Paleo, beans are replaced with white potatoes.

PREP TIME: 10 MINUTES
COOK TIME: 4–8 HOURS

INGREDIENTS | SERVES 6

2 pounds ground pork

¼ cup ghee

½ teaspoon ground cumin

½ teaspoon sea salt

1 large onion, peeled and chopped

2 (4") jalapeños, stemmed and quartered

3 cloves garlic, peeled and chopped

10 cups Chicken Stock (see recipe in this chapter)

3 large white potatoes, peeled and chopped

1. In a large skillet over medium-high heat, cook pork in ghee with cumin, salt, and onion until fully cooked, about 7–10 minutes.

2. Add pork mixture to a 6-quart slow cooker along with remaining ingredients. Cover and cook on low heat 8 hours or on high heat 4 hours.

Per Serving   Calories: 508 | Fat: 23g | Protein: 41g | Sodium: 1,116mg | Fiber: 4g | Carbohydrates: 34g | Sugar: 3.5g

Any White Meat

This chili recipe works with any white meat, including ground chicken or turkey. Additionally, swap shredded meat for ground meat for a thicker stew.

Slow-Cooker Fish Stew

Bring fresh coastal flavors to your kitchen with this hearty fish stew.

PREP TIME: 10 MINUTES
COOK TIME: 25–30 MINUTES

INGREDIENTS | SERVES 6

4 cups Fish Stock (see recipe in this chapter)

2 large red bell peppers, seeded and chopped

6 medium yellow potatoes, peeled and chopped

1 medium onion, peeled and chopped

2 medium stalks celery, chopped

2 tablespoons Worcestershire sauce

4 cloves garlic, peeled and chopped

1 teaspoon sea salt

¼ teaspoon ground black pepper

4 (6-ounce) cod fillets

1 pound raw medium shrimp, peeled and deveined

1. In a large stockpot over medium-high heat, combine all ingredients except cod and shrimp. Bring to a boil, reduce heat, and simmer 15 minutes.

2. While mixture is simmering, rinse fish and shrimp and pat dry with paper towels. Cut cod into ½" pieces.

3. Add cod and shrimp to stockpot and stir; cook over medium-low heat 5–7 minutes or until cod flakes easily with a fork. Do not overcook.

Per Serving Calories: 317 | Fat: 2g | Protein: 35g | Sodium: 989mg | Fiber: 6g | Carbohydrates: 37g | Sugar: 7g

Something's Fishy Here

Any whitefish will work for this recipe, including halibut or tilapia, or any combination. For a flavor swap, try using chicken stock instead of fish stock.

Slow-Cooker Beef Bone Broth

Bone broth is all the rage right now, and for good reason: It's rich in minerals, collagen, and even protein that nourish the body right down to tendons, joints, and bones.

PREP TIME: 1 HOUR
COOK TIME: 14–26 HOURS

INGREDIENTS | MAKES 10 CUPS

2 pounds beef soup bones (including marrow)

10 cups water

2 large carrots, peeled and halved

2 large onions, peeled and quartered

2 medium stalks celery, halved

2 cloves garlic, peeled and quartered

2 teaspoons sea salt

1 teaspoon ground black pepper

2 tablespoons apple cider vinegar

Them Bones, Them Bones

You can often get bones for free from local meat markets or butchers, especially if you purchase meat in bulk. Don't forget to ask for the marrow, too!

1. In an 8-quart slow cooker, combine all ingredients, cover, and cook on high heat 4–6 hours. Reduce heat to low and cook an additional 10–20 hours.

2. Let broth cool about 1 hour, and remove bones and large vegetable chunks while still warm. Strain broth through cheesecloth to remove all particles.

3. As the broth cools to room temperature, the fat will separate to the top. Do not discard the fat. Place broth in airtight containers. Can be refrigerated up to 4 days, or frozen up to 6 months. The solidified fat will return to liquid form when it is reheated.

Per Serving (1 cup) Calories: 63 | Fat: 5g | Protein: 4g | Sodium: 492mg | Fiber: 0.3g | Carbohydrates: 1g | Sugar: 0.3g

Slow-Cooker Chicken Bone Broth

This alternative to beef bone broth is just as nourishing, and perfect for a nutrient-packed addition to chicken soups, or for sipping on its own when you're feeling under the weather.

PREP TIME: 1 HOUR
COOK TIME: 10–18 HOURS

INGREDIENTS | MAKES 10 CUPS

3 pounds chicken pieces (including neck)
3 medium stalks celery, halved
3 large carrots, peeled and halved
1 large onion, peeled and quartered
3 cloves garlic, peeled and quartered
2 small Granny Smith apples, quartered
2 teaspoons sea salt
¼ teaspoon ground black pepper
1 teaspoon dried thyme
9 cups water
2 tablespoons apple cider vinegar

1. In an 8-quart slow cooker, add all ingredients, cover, and cook on high heat 4–6 hours. Reduce heat to low and cook an additional 6–12 hours.

2. Allow broth to cool about 1 hour, and remove chicken pieces and vegetables while still warm. Strain broth through cheesecloth to remove all particles.

3. Pour broth into airtight containers and cover. Refrigerate up to 3 days or freeze up to 6 months.

Per Serving (1 cup) Calories: 47 | Fat: 4g | Protein: 1.5g | Sodium: 498mg | Fiber: 0.4g | Carbohydrates: 2g | Sugar: 1g

Fish Stock

Use this stock in any fish or seafood dish instead of water or chicken stock.

PREP TIME: 12 HOURS
COOK TIME: 8–10 HOURS

INGREDIENTS | MAKES 3 QUARTS

3 quarts water
2 large onions, peeled and quartered
Head and bones of 3 fish, any type
2 medium stalks celery, chopped
2 tablespoons peppercorns
1 bunch parsley

1. Place all ingredients in a 4-quart slow cooker. Cover and cook on low 8–10 hours.

2. Remove all solids. Transfer to an airtight container. Refrigerate overnight.

3. The next day, skim off any foam that has floated to the top. Refrigerate and use within 1 week or freeze up to 3 months.

Per Serving (1 cup) Calories: 24 | Fat: 1g | Protein: 1.5g | Sodium: 23mg | Fiber: 0.5g | Carbohydrates: 2.5g | Sugar: 1g

Chicken Stock

This classic kitchen staple is a simple yet tasty base for soups and stews.

PREP TIME: 10 MINUTES
COOK TIME: 2–3 HOURS

INGREDIENTS | MAKES 10 CUPS

6 pounds chicken parts (whole bird or bone-in pieces, including necks, feet, and backs)

2 large onions, peeled and quartered

3 large carrots, peeled and halved

2 medium stalks celery, halved

1 medium leek, trimmed and halved

3 cloves garlic, peeled and quartered

2 teaspoons dried thyme

1 teaspoon dried rosemary

2 teaspoons sea salt

½ teaspoon ground black pepper

15 cups water

1. In a large stockpot over medium-high heat, add all ingredients and cover with water. Bring to a boil, reduce heat to medium-low, and simmer uncovered 2–3 hours.

2. Using a slotted spoon, remove all solid chunks.

3. Strain broth through cheesecloth or a fine sieve and store in airtight containers in refrigerator up to 3 days or freezer up to 6 months.

Per Serving (1 cup) Calories: 62 | Fat: 4g | Protein: 3g | Sodium: 488mg | Fiber: 1g | Carbohydrates: 2g | Sugar: 1g

Beef Stock

This classic beef stock is the perfect base for any red meat soup or stew, including beef, lamb, and bison.

PREP TIME: 10 MINUTES
COOK TIME: 6–8 HOURS

INGREDIENTS | MAKES 10 CUPS

6 pounds beef soup bones

1 large onion, peeled and quartered

3 large carrots, peeled and halved

2 medium stalks celery, halved

4 medium Roma tomatoes, halved

1 medium parsnip, peeled and chopped

1 white potato, peeled and chopped

½ tablespoon ground black pepper

½ tablespoon sea salt

2 teaspoons dried thyme

4 cloves garlic, peeled and quartered

15 cups water

1. In a large stockpot over medium-high heat, add all ingredients and cover with water. Bring to a boil, reduce heat to medium-low, and simmer uncovered 6–8 hours.

2. Using a slotted spoon, remove all solid chunks.

3. Strain broth through cheesecloth or a fine sieve and store in airtight containers in the refrigerator up to 3 days or the freezer up to 6 months.

Per Serving (1 cup) Calories: 93 | Fat: 6.5g | Protein: 5g | Sodium: 502.5mg | Fiber: 0.4g | Carbohydrates: 4g | Sugar: 1g

Turkey Stock

Popular during the holidays, this is the perfect way to put your leftover turkey to good use. This can also be used as a substitute in recipes that call for chicken stock.

PREP TIME: 3–5 HOURS
COOK TIME: 6–8 HOURS

INGREDIENTS | YIELDS 1 GALLON

10 black peppercorns

6 sprigs parsley

4 medium carrots, peeled and thickly sliced

4 stalks celery, thickly sliced

1 gallon water

2 medium onions, peeled and thickly sliced

2 leeks (white parts only), thickly sliced

1 turkey carcass, cut up

1½ teaspoons dried thyme

1 teaspoon pepper

1. Combine all ingredients except pepper in a 6-quart slow cooker. Cover and cook on low 6–8 hours.

2. Strain stock through a double-layer of cheesecloth, discarding solids. Season with pepper.

3. Refrigerate 3–5 hours until chilled. Remove fat from surface of stock.

4. Freeze or refrigerate stock and use within 1 week or freeze up to 3 months.

Per Serving (1 cup) Calories: 27 | Fat: 1g | Protein: 3g | Sodium: 90mg | Fiber: 0.3g | Carbohydrates: 1g | Sugar: 0.5g

Basic Vegetable Stock

This stock is low in sodium and high in disease-fighting phytochemicals. Try adding mushrooms for additional flavor.

PREP TIME: 15 MINUTES
COOK TIME: 2 HOURS 15 MINUTES

INGREDIENTS | MAKES 1 GALLON

2 pounds yellow onions, peeled and roughly chopped

1 pound carrots, peeled and roughly chopped

1 pound celery, stalks roughly chopped

1 bunch fresh parsley stems, roughly chopped

1½ gallons water

4 sprigs fresh thyme

2 bay leaves (fresh or dried)

10–20 peppercorns

1. Place vegetables, parsley, and water in a stockpot over medium heat; bring to a simmer and cook uncovered 1½ hours.

2. Add herbs and peppercorns and continue to simmer uncovered 45 minutes.

3. Strain broth through cheesecloth or a fine sieve and store in airtight containers in the refrigerator up to 3 days or the freezer up to 6 months.

Per Serving (1 cup) Calories: 7 | Fat: 0.1g | Protein: 0.3g | Sodium: 11mg | Fiber: 0.7g | Carbohydrates: 2g | Sugar: 0.5g

CHAPTER 7

Paleo Fats

Old-Fashioned Paleo Biscuits

These melt-in-your-mouth biscuits work well paired with just about anything (gravy, stew, honey, etc.) and can be used for both savory meals and desserts (Paleo strawberry shortcake, anyone?). Don't fear the lard, because it's the secret to making these biscuits truly divine.

PREP TIME: 20 MINUTES
COOK TIME: 15–18 MINUTES

INGREDIENTS | SERVES 10

2½ cups cassava flour
1½ teaspoons baking soda
1½ teaspoons cream of tartar
½ teaspoon fine sea salt
⅓ cup lard, cold
1 cup full-fat coconut milk
1 tablespoon ghee

Spotlight on Lard

In the early and mid-twentieth century, lard was a staple cooking fat because of its wide availability—people butchered their own pigs and used every part of them, which included rendering their own lard for cooking. Lard is also a good dietary source of vitamin D, which is essential for optimal wellness and thyroid function.

1. Preheat oven to 400°F. Line a baking sheet with parchment paper.

2. In a large mixing bowl, combine flour, baking soda, cream of tartar, and salt. Cut lard into flour mixture using a fork until it resembles large crumbs. Add coconut milk and stir just until combined.

3. Using wet hands, form dough into 10 equal-sized balls and place on prepared baking sheet. Flatten biscuits using a spoon until about 1" thick. Use a basting brush to coat biscuits with ghee.

4. Bake 15–18 minutes or until biscuits are golden brown and the center is not doughy when poked with a knife. Let cool 5 minutes before serving. Keep in refrigerator up to 3 days.

Per Serving (1 biscuit) Calories: 235 | Fat: 14g | Protein: 1g | Sodium: 303mg | Fiber: 2g | Carbohydrates: 29g | Sugar: 0.4g

Tallow-Roasted Bok Choy

This simple roasted vegetable dish can be thrown together in just a few minutes and makes the perfect addition to any protein dish for breakfast, lunch, or dinner.

PREP TIME: 5 MINUTES
COOK TIME: 10–13 MINUTES

INGREDIENTS | SERVES 4

3 cloves garlic, peeled and smashed

2 tablespoons tallow

10 heads baby bok choy, cut into 1" pieces

1 teaspoon fine sea salt

In a large skillet over medium-high heat sauté garlic in tallow until it turns slightly brown, about 3 minutes. Add bok choy and salt and sauté 7–10 minutes or until bok choy starts to soften and wilt, stirring frequently to ensure even cooking and coating with the tallow. Serve warm.

Per Serving   Calories: 99 | Fat: 6.5g | Protein: 4g | Sodium: 774mg | Fiber: 3g | Carbohydrates: 7g | Sugar: 3g

Spotlight on Tallow

Tallow, that is rendered from beef suet, is a Paleo superfood because it's rich in antioxidants such as vitamins A and E and contains anti-inflammatory and anti-microbial fatty acids that are perfect for nourishing your body's cells, preventing cancer, and preventing premature aging.

Coconut Fried Sweet Potatoes

The coconut oil brings out the already sweet profile of the potatoes, and the addition of some coconut sugar further expands the coconut goodness that this delectable side dish provides.

PREP TIME: 5 MINUTES
COOK TIME: 12–15 MINUTES

INGREDIENTS | SERVES 4

4 medium sweet potatoes, peeled and finely chopped

3 tablespoons coconut oil

2 tablespoons coconut sugar

½ teaspoon fine sea salt

In a large skillet over medium-high heat combine all ingredients. Sauté until potatoes begin to blacken around the edges, about 12–15 minutes. Stir frequently to ensure even cooking. Serve warm.

Per Serving   Calories: 257 | Fat: 10g | Protein: 3g | Sodium: 338mg | Fiber: 5g | Carbohydrates: 40g | Sugar: 17g

Spotlight on Coconut Oil

Coconut oil's clear color and ability to be absorbed well into the skin makes coconut oil the perfect moisturizer, face wash, hair mask, cuticle softener, diaper rash protectant, mouthwash, and more.

"Buttery" Baked Chicken

The benefit of baking chicken with ghee is that the meat stays moist and tender while bringing out the decadent and rich flavors that you get when you cook with butter. The addition of herbs gives the meat a nice flavor profile that pairs nicely with root vegetables or as a topping on a salad.

PREP TIME: 5 MINUTES
COOK TIME: 12–15 MINUTES

INGREDIENTS | SERVES 4

4 (6-ounce) boneless, skinless chicken breasts
¼ cup ghee
1 teaspoon dried rosemary
1 teaspoon dried thyme
1 teaspoon fine sea salt
1 teaspoon onion powder
1 teaspoon garlic powder
2 medium lemons, juiced

1. Preheat oven to 400°F. Lay chicken breasts in a large glass baking pan.

2. In a small mixing bowl, combine remaining ingredients. Brush chicken with spice mixture and pour remaining liquid into the baking pan.

3. Bake chicken 12–15 minutes or until the center of the chicken reads 165°F on a meat thermometer. Do not overcook. Serve warm.

Per Serving Calories: 399 | Fat: 20g | Protein: 52g | Sodium: 648mg | Fiber: 0.3g | Carbohydrates: 2g | Sugar: 0.4g

Spotlight on Ghee

Ghee, which is butter that has been cooked to remove milk solids, is a popular Paleo fat that gives foods the richness of dairy without any of the possible cross-reactivity that can happen for people with dietary issues or sensitivities. Ghee is an excellent source of the fat-soluble vitamins A and E, both of which have antioxidant properties within the body.

Paleo Guacamole

This spicy guacamole is sure to be a hit at any party, or as the topping to an epic plate of Paleo-friendly cheese-less nachos or tacos. It also pairs well with vegetable sticks and Paleo crackers.

PREP TIME: 30 MINUTES
COOK TIME: N/A

INGREDIENTS | SERVES 4

4 medium ripe avocados, pitted and peeled

1 medium green bell pepper, seeded and diced

1 medium red bell pepper, seeded and diced

2 teaspoons garlic powder

1 teaspoon onion powder

1 teaspoon chili powder

½ teaspoon fine sea salt

¼ teaspoon ground black pepper

⅛ teaspoon red pepper flakes

2 teaspoons avocado oil

1 (500-milligram) vitamin C tablet, crushed

1 small white onion, peeled and diced

In a food processor or blender, purée avocado until smooth. Stir in remaining ingredients by hand. Chill in refrigerator before serving.

Per Serving Calories: 277 | Fat: 21g | Protein: 4g | Sodium: 313mg | Fiber: 11g | Carbohydrates: 19g | Sugar: 3g

Spotlight on Avocado

Like many Paleo fats, avocado is rich in omega-3 fatty acids, but it's also an excellent dietary source of vitamin K and folate—both nutrients that are vital for healthy blood, energy production within the body, and consequently, thyroid function. An avocado a day could be as beneficial for doctor avoidance as the proverbial apple a day.

Sautéed Mushrooms with Garlic

Perhaps one of the most underused Paleo fats, duck fat is sublime because its ultra-smooth taste blends better with savory dishes than the sweeter-tasting and more frequently used coconut oil. It is also more than 50 percent monounsaturated fat, and remains more stable at higher cooking temperatures.

PREP TIME: 5 MINUTES
COOK TIME: 7 MINUTES

INGREDIENTS | SERVES 4

2 pounds portobello mushrooms, quartered

2 tablespoons duck fat

½ teaspoon fine sea salt

¼ teaspoon ground black pepper

1 clove garlic, peeled and chopped

In a large skillet over medium-high heat, combine all ingredients and sauté until mushrooms are soft and spongy, about 7 minutes. Stir frequently to avoid overcooking on one side. Serve warm as a side dish or appetizer.

Per Serving   Calories: 109 | Fat: 6.5g | Protein: 5g | Sodium: 300mg | Fiber: 3g | Carbohydrates: 9g | Sugar: 6g

Spotlight on Duck Fat

Even though you don't have to be afraid of saturated fats, varying the types of fat you eat provides greater health benefits. Duck fat is rich in monounsaturated fats and is rich in linoleic acid, an EFA (essential fatty acid) that supports healthy kidney function and boosts the energy-producing centers of your body's cells.

Ginger Baked Salmon

This fatty fish is the ultimate in anti-inflammatory eating, and this zesty recipe pairs the warmth of ginger with the zest of lemon, all culminating in a melt-in-your-mouth meal that'll have you singing the praises of this superfood.

PREP TIME: 10 MINUTES
COOK TIME: 18–20 MINUTES

INGREDIENTS | SERVES 4

4 (½-pound) wild-caught salmon fillets
1 large lemon, zested and juiced
1 large orange, zested and juiced
¼ cup ghee
1 teaspoon fine sea salt
¼ teaspoon black pepper
1 tablespoon freshly grated ginger

Spotlight on Salmon

One of the few dietary sources rich in vitamin D, salmon is also an excellent source of vitamin B$_{12}$ and selenium. All three are critical nutrients for proper thyroid function, so making salmon a regular part of your Hashimoto's Paleo diet will go a long way in promoting healing and hormone balance.

1. Preheat oven to 425°F. If fish is frozen, ensure that it is thoroughly thawed before cooking.

2. On a baking sheet, lay salmon fillets so that they aren't touching. In a small mixing bowl, combine remaining ingredients and stir. Using a basting brush or a spoon, evenly coat each fillet with the mixture.

3. Bake 18–20 minutes (slightly longer depending on the thickness of the cut) until the center of the salmon flakes easily with a fork. The center should still be dark pink for that melt-in-your-mouth texture. Serve warm.

Per Serving Calories: 471 | Fat: 28g | Protein: 45g | Sodium: 659mg | Fiber: 0.1g | Carbohydrates: 2.5g | Sugar: 1.5g

Fried Sardines

There are not many fried items in a Paleo diet, because most fried dishes are made with flour. This is a healthier alternative to traditional frying. The alcohol in the wine is mostly cooked off, so you will not have to worry about the alcohol either.

PREP TIME: 5 MINUTES
COOK TIME: 25 MINUTES

INGREDIENTS | SERVES 6

1 cup almond flour

2 pounds boneless, skinless, no-salt-added sardines

¾ cup plus 1 tablespoon almond oil, divided

2 cloves garlic, peeled and chopped

1 cup dry white wine

1 cup apple cider vinegar

½ cup chopped mint leaves

Spotlight on Sardines

Even though people are often grossed out by these tiny fish, they're one of the most nutrient-dense fish available. One 3-ounce serving of sardines contains more than 300 percent daily value of vitamin B_{12}, and they're also rich in selenium, vitamin D, and copper—all essential nutrients required for production of thyroid hormone.

1. Pour flour into a shallow dish. Roll sardines in flour.

2. Heat ¾ cup oil in a large frying pan over medium-high heat.

3. When oil is hot, fry sardines until brown and crispy, about 5 minutes. Drain on paper towels and keep warm.

4. In another frying pan over medium heat, warm garlic in remaining 1 tablespoon oil. Cook 1 minute.

5. Add wine and vinegar. Simmer mixture, stirring occasionally, until reduced by half, about 15 minutes.

6. Pour sauce over sardines and sprinkle with fresh mint.

Per Serving Calories: 526 | Fat: 34g | Protein: 39g | Sodium: 105mg | Fiber: 2g | Carbohydrates: 6g | Sugar: 1g

Olive Oil–Braised Brussels Sprouts with Apples

This sweet and savory side dish pairs perfectly with chicken, pork, or turkey for any meal of the day.

PREP TIME: 10 MINUTES
COOK TIME: 30–35 MINUTES

INGREDIENTS | SERVES 4

⅓ cup extra-virgin olive oil

1 large lemon, peeled and juiced (save the peel)

2 tablespoons apple cider vinegar

3 cloves garlic, peeled and chopped

1 teaspoon fine sea salt

4 cups Brussels sprouts, trimmed and halved

2 large Granny Smith apples, sliced

1 tablespoon raw honey

1. Preheat oven to 400°F.

2. In a large mixing bowl, toss all ingredients together (including lemon peel) and spread evenly on a baking sheet. Bake 30–35 minutes or until the outer leaves of Brussels sprouts turn dark brown and curl up from crispness. Serve warm or chilled. Refrigerate up to 3 days.

Per Serving   Calories: 253 | Fat: 14g | Protein: 4g | Sodium: 583mg | Fiber: 6g | Carbohydrates: 27.5g | Sugar: 16g

Spotlight on Olive Oil

Perhaps the most long-standing fat associated with anti-inflammatory health benefits, olive oil is rich in polyphenols that can reduce the risk of heart disease, as well as autoimmune processes within the body.

CHAPTER 8

Breakfast

Toasted Nut "Cereal"

Cereal is an easy weekday breakfast. But packaged products are loaded with sweeteners, preservatives, and artificial colors. Make your own "cereal" and you won't miss the packaged stuff at all.

PREP TIME: 45 MINUTES
COOK TIME: 25–35 MINUTES

INGREDIENTS | MAKES 10 CUPS

1½ cups pumpkin seeds
1 cup sunflower seeds
1½ cups sliced almonds
1½ cups chopped pecans
1½ cups unsweetened coconut flakes
⅓ cup Grade B maple syrup
⅓ cup coconut oil
1 teaspoon ground cinnamon
2 teaspoons vanilla extract
1 cup dried cranberries
1 cup chopped dried apricots
1 cup golden raisins

1. Preheat oven to 375°F. Line a rimmed baking sheet with parchment paper and set aside.

2. In a large bowl, combine pumpkin seeds, sunflower seeds, almonds, pecans, and coconut. Pour mixture onto lined baking sheet.

3. In a small saucepan, combine maple syrup and coconut oil and heat gently until coconut oil is melted. Remove from heat and stir in cinnamon and vanilla. Drizzle over the mixture on baking sheet and toss to coat. Spread evenly.

4. Bake 20–30 minutes, stirring every 10 minutes, until light golden brown and fragrant. Remove from oven and stir in cranberries, apricots, and raisins. Let stand until cool, stirring occasionally. Store in an airtight container at room temperature.

Per Serving (½ cup)   Calories: 270 | Fat: 18.5g | Protein: 6.5g | Sodium: 3mg | Fiber: 4g | Carbohydrates: 22g | Sugar: 14g

Coconut Muesli

Muesli is typically a mixture of raw oats, seeds, nuts, and dried fruit. But here's a surprise: You don't need the oatmeal! Coconut flakes make a flavorful substitute. Plus, they're filled with fiber and healthy fat.

PREP TIME: 10 MINUTES
COOK TIME: N/A

INGREDIENTS | SERVES 8

2 cups unsweetened coconut flakes

2 cups slivered almonds

1 cup chopped macadamia nuts

1 cup broken walnuts

½ cup sesame seeds

½ cup pumpkin seeds

1 cup golden raisins

1 cup dried unsweetened cranberries

1 cup chopped Medjool dates

1 teaspoon ground cinnamon

1 teaspoon ground ginger

½ teaspoon ground nutmeg

8 cups unsweetened almond or hazelnut milk

1. In a large bowl, combine all ingredients except milk and mix well. Store in an airtight container at room temperature.

2. To serve, pour 1 cup muesli into a bowl and add 1 cup almond or hazelnut milk. Let stand 5 minutes before eating.

3. You can also make this muesli the night before. Place muesli in a large bowl and cover with milk. Cover and let stand overnight in the refrigerator. When you're ready to eat breakfast, stir the muesli and dig in.

Per Serving (1 cup muesli and 1 cup unsweetened almond milk) Calories: 702 | Fat: 55g | Protein: 16g | Sodium: 23.5mg | Fiber: 13g | Carbohydrates: 45g | Sugar: 23.5g

Crunchy Muesli

For crunchier muesli, toast the coconut flakes, nuts, and seeds. Spread on a baking sheet and bake at 350°F 10–15 minutes until fragrant and light brown. Let cool before combining with remaining ingredients.

Sweet Potato Chia Pudding

This sweet and savory AIP-compliant breakfast pudding can easily be customized to personal taste preferences with the addition of toppings, and as a bonus, it can also double as a dessert!

PREP TIME: 4–6 HOURS
COOK TIME: 15 MINUTES

INGREDIENTS | SERVES 4

1 small sweet potato, peeled
2 cups water
2 tablespoons unsweetened coconut flakes
1 cup full-fat coconut milk
1 teaspoon vanilla extract
1 teaspoon ground cinnamon
2 tablespoons unsweetened applesauce
¼ cup chia seeds

1. In a small saucepan over medium heat, boil sweet potato in water until soft and easily mashed with a fork. Remove from heat and let cool.

2. In a food processor or blender, purée sweet potato with coconut flakes, coconut milk, vanilla, cinnamon, and applesauce until thoroughly combined and smooth.

3. Stir chia seeds into mixture and refrigerate 4–6 hours. Serve chilled. Keep in refrigerator up to 2 days.

Per Serving   Calories: 172 | Fat: 15g | Protein: 3g | Sodium: 16mg | Fiber: 3g | Carbohydrates: 8g | Sugar: 2g

Chia N'oatmeal

Missing oats on a Paleo diet? This breakfast dish is reminiscent of the classic warm breakfast cereal and will satisfy that comfort craving at any time of the day. Change up the flavor by using different fruit and nut butters.

PREP TIME: 4–12 HOURS
COOK TIME: 10 MINUTES (OPTIONAL)

INGREDIENTS | SERVES 2

2 tablespoons chia seeds
1 tablespoon hemp protein powder
10 ounces full-fat coconut milk
1 teaspoon ground cinnamon
¼ teaspoon ground nutmeg
2 teaspoons Grade B maple syrup
1 large ripe banana, peeled
1 tablespoon unsweetened almond butter

1. In a medium mixing bowl stir together chia seeds, hemp powder, and coconut milk. Refrigerate 4–6 hours or overnight to allow chia seeds to absorb liquid.

2. In a food processor or blender, combine chia mixture with remaining ingredients. Pulse until well combined.

3. Optional: heat in a small saucepan over medium-low heat until warmed, about 10 minutes.

Per Serving   Calories: 450 | Fat: 35g | Protein: 8g | Sodium: 44mg | Fiber: 6.5g | Carbohydrates: 30g | Sugar: 13g

Chicken and "Grits"

This Paleo take on a classic southern dish offers a filling breakfast meal that can also double as a dinner.

PREP TIME: 15 MINUTES
COOK TIME: 40 MINUTES

INGREDIENTS | SERVES 4

4 (5-ounce) boneless, skinless chicken breasts
½ cup ghee, divided
2 teaspoons sea salt, divided
1 teaspoon ground black pepper, divided
3 large turnips, peeled and quartered
7 cups Chicken Stock, divided (see recipe in Chapter 6)
1 teaspoon garlic powder
½ cup bacon crumbles

1. Preheat oven to 375°F. Place chicken in a 9" × 13" baking pan and coat with ¼ cup ghee. Sprinkle with 1 teaspoon salt and ½ teaspoon pepper. Bake 20 minutes or until chicken is cooked in the center. (Internal temperature should read 165°F on a meat thermometer.)

2. Meanwhile, in a large stockpot, boil turnips in 6 cups stock until soft in the center, about 20 minutes. Remove from heat and drain stock.

3. Using a food processor, blender, or potato masher, pulse or mash turnips and then stir in remaining salt, pepper, and stock. Add garlic powder and bacon crumbles, and stir once more until well combined. Top chicken with mashed turnips and serve warm.

Per Serving Calories: 707 | Fat: 46g | Protein: 53g | Sodium: 2,517mg | Fiber: 2.5g | Carbohydrates: 10g | Sugar: 4.5g

Breakfast Root Medley

This AIP-friendly breakfast is both savory and satisfying,
and can be cooked ahead of time for easy breakfasts all week long.

PREP TIME: 10 MINUTES
COOK TIME: 45 MINUTES

INGREDIENTS | SERVES 6

1 large beet, peeled and sliced

1 teaspoon fine sea salt, divided

4 tablespoons ghee, divided

2 large sweet potatoes, peeled and spiralized

1 large turnip, peeled and spiralized

1 large parsnip, peeled and spiralized

1 small onion, peeled and diced

2 large zucchini, spiralized

2 small apples, cored and spiralized

Egg-Less

AIP meals don't include eggs since they can often be problematic for people with autoimmune issues or leaky gut. If you know you're not sensitive to eggs, you can serve this root medley on a bed of scrambled or over-medium eggs for some added fat and protein.

1. Preheat oven to 400°F. Spread beet slices across a baking sheet. In a small mixing bowl stir together half of salt and half of ghee. Spread mixture across beet slices. Bake 20 minutes or until beets are soft.

2. In a large skillet over medium-high heat, add remaining salt and ghee, along with sweet potatoes, turnip, parsnip, and onion. Sauté until softened, about 10 minutes, stirring frequently. Reduce heat to medium and add zucchini and apple; cook another 3–5 minutes, stirring frequently.

3. Add medley to baking sheet on top of beets and bake 5–7 minutes or until vegetables begin to brown.

4. Remove from heat and serve warm.

Per Serving Calories: 175 | Fat: 8g | Protein: 3g | Sodium: 328mg | Fiber: 5g | Carbohydrates: 24g | Sugar: 12g

Apple Spice Chia Pudding

This spiced breakfast pudding is filling and decadent while packed with antioxidants and other good-for-you nutrients. It's a breakfast win-win!

PREP TIME: 4–6 HOURS
COOK TIME: N/A

INGREDIENTS | SERVES 2

1 cup unsweetened almond milk

1 cup full-fat coconut milk

1 tablespoon chia seeds

1 small Golden Delicious apple, peeled, cored, and sliced

2 pitted Medjool dates

½ teaspoon ground cinnamon

¼ teaspoon ground nutmeg

1 tablespoon raw honey

2 tablespoons raw cacao nibs

1. In a medium bowl, combine milks and chia seeds. Cover and let sit in refrigerator 4–6 hours so chia seeds soak up liquid.

2. In a food processor or blender, add chia seed mixture with apple, dates, cinnamon, nutmeg, and honey. Pulse until smooth. Serve chilled, topped with cacao nibs.

Per Serving   Calories: 444 | Fat: 29.5g | Protein: 4g | Sodium: 94mg | Fiber: 5g | Carbohydrates: 43g | Sugar: 31g

Ham and Parsnip Breakfast Hash

This twist on meat and potatoes for breakfast gives all the comforts of breakfast flavors with the added bonus of being AIP-friendly and egg-free.

PREP TIME: 5 MINUTES
COOK TIME: 18–22 MINUTES

INGREDIENTS | SERVES 4

3 large parsnips, peeled and chopped

4 tablespoons ghee, divided

2 pounds ham, cubed

½ teaspoon sea salt

4 cloves garlic, peeled and chopped

1 small white onion, peeled and diced

2 tablespoons unsweetened applesauce

In a large skillet over medium heat, cook parsnips in 2 tablespoons ghee until they begin to soften, about 8–10 minutes. Add remaining ingredients and cook 10–12 minutes until ham is fully browned. Serve warm.

Per Serving   Calories: 632 | Fat: 37g | Protein: 39g | Sodium: 2,657mg | Fiber: 5g | Carbohydrates: 31g | Sugar: 6g

Farm-Style Egg Skillet

All the familiar flavors of a diner-cooked breakfast, easily thrown together at home!

PREP TIME: 10 MINUTES
COOK TIME: 30 MINUTES

INGREDIENTS | SERVES 4

8 strips bacon

1 tablespoon ghee

3 large white potatoes, peeled and shredded

½ pound white mushrooms, halved

2 cups baby spinach

1 large green bell pepper, seeded and chopped

1 large red bell pepper, seeded and chopped

1 small yellow onion, peeled and chopped

½ teaspoon garlic powder

½ teaspoon onion powder

½ teaspoon fine sea salt

½ teaspoon ground black pepper

4 large eggs

1. In a large skillet over medium heat, cook bacon until browned, about 5 minutes per side. Set aside, leaving bacon drippings in pan. Add ghee and potatoes and sauté until potatoes begin to brown, about 7 minutes.

2. Cut bacon into ½" pieces and add to potatoes in skillet. Stir in mushrooms, spinach, bell peppers, onion, garlic powder, onion powder, salt, and pepper. Sauté until vegetables are softened, about 10 minutes. Make four wells in the vegetable mixture and crack an egg into each well. Cook over medium heat until eggs are cooked to desired doneness. Serve warm.

Per Serving Calories: 435 | Fat: 16g | Protein: 22g | Sodium: 766mg | Fiber: 6g | Carbohydrates: 50g | Sugar: 6g

Save That Fat!

Bacon drippings are a nutritious and tasty fat that can be used to flavor your dishes, make salad dressings, and even cook other meats. Even if you're not using them for the dish you're cooking, save them for later in a glass jar in the refrigerator. But whatever you do, don't ever throw them out!

Chicken Bacon Skillet

This yummy one-pan breakfast can double as lunch or dinner, too.
Change up the recipe by varying the kinds of vegetables used.

PREP TIME: 5 MINUTES
COOK TIME: 17–20 MINUTES

INGREDIENTS | SERVES 4

10 slices bacon, cut into 1" pieces

1 pound ground chicken

½ teaspoon sea salt

½ teaspoon ground black pepper

1 cup Chicken Stock (see recipe in Chapter 6)

1 bunch asparagus, trimmed

1 bunch broccoli, cut into florets

2 tablespoons ghee

1 teaspoon onion powder

1. In a large skillet over medium heat cook bacon, chicken, salt, pepper, and stock until chicken is fully cooked and no pink is visible, about 10 minutes. Stir frequently.

2. Add asparagus, broccoli, ghee, and onion powder to skillet. Cover and let cook until asparagus begins to soften, about 7–10 minutes, stirring every few minutes. Serve warm.

Per Serving Calories: 472 | Fat: 30g | Protein: 40g | Sodium: 1,012mg | Fiber: 3.5g | Carbohydrates: 9g | Sugar: 2.5g

Bacon and Vegetable Omelet

Bacon and eggs are a breakfast tradition and they are 100 percent Paleo-approved.

PREP TIME: 5 MINUTES
COOK TIME: 30 MINUTES

INGREDIENTS | SERVES 2

6 slices bacon, diced

1 medium yellow summer squash, chopped

1 cup sliced mushrooms

1 medium zucchini, chopped

¼ cup chopped fresh basil leaves

2 tablespoons olive oil

8 large eggs, beaten

1. In a large sauté pan, cook bacon until crispy, about 8 minutes. Add vegetables and basil to pan and sauté until tender, about 5–8 minutes.

2. Meanwhile, heat olive oil in a second sauté pan over medium heat.

3. Cook eggs until almost set, about 3-5 minutes.

4. Place vegetable and bacon mixture along one side of omelet and fold other half over to enclose filling. Serve.

Per Serving Calories: 602 | Fat: 42.5g | Protein: 40g | Sodium: 873mg | Fiber: 2g | Carbohydrates: 9g | Sugar: 6g

Sweet Potato and Egg Skillet

This meal is so filling that it'll keep you full for hours, and the warming combination of sweet potatoes, onion, and spinach will have you planning this meal for dinnertime, too.

PREP TIME: 5 MINUTES
COOK TIME: 15 MINUTES

INGREDIENTS | SERVES 4

8 large eggs
½ cup unsweetened almond milk
3 tablespoons ghee, divided
¼ teaspoon ground cumin
¼ teaspoon garlic powder
¼ teaspoon onion powder
½ teaspoon fine sea salt
¼ teaspoon ground black pepper
2 large sweet potatoes, sliced into ½" pieces
2 green onions, sliced
3 cups baby spinach

1. In a medium mixing bowl, whisk eggs with milk, 1 tablespoon ghee, cumin, garlic powder, onion powder, salt, and pepper. Set aside.

2. In a large skillet over medium heat add remaining ghee, potatoes, and onions. Cook 8–10 minutes until potatoes soften, stirring frequently.

3. Add spinach to skillet and cook an additional 1–2 minutes until leaves wilt. Pour egg mixture into skillet and continue to cook 2–3 minutes, stirring occasionally so the egg cooks evenly. When egg is cooked to desired doneness, remove from heat and serve immediately.

Per Serving   Calories: 322 | Fat: 20g | Protein: 15g | Sodium: 485mg | Fiber: 3g | Carbohydrates: 17g | Sugar: 5g

Spanish Eggs

This spicy breakfast is sure to wake you up in the morning!

PREP TIME: 5 MINUTES
COOK TIME: 15 MINUTES

INGREDIENTS | SERVES 4

2 tablespoons coconut oil

1 medium onion, peeled and chopped

2 cloves garlic, peeled and chopped

4 large tomatoes, chopped

2 small zucchini, sliced

½ teaspoon sea salt

5 large eggs

1 teaspoon onion powder

1 teaspoon chili powder

2 large avocados, peeled, pitted, and sliced

1. Heat oil in a large skillet over medium-high heat and add onion and garlic. Sauté 3–5 minutes until onion starts to caramelize. Reduce heat to medium and add tomatoes, zucchini, and salt. Stir frequently and cook an additional 5 minutes.

2. Crack eggs over skillet mixture (or in a separate bowl, if preferred, and pour over skillet) and add onion and chili powders. Stir all together and cook until eggs are still moist but the whites are firm, 5–8 minutes.

3. Remove from heat, portion out into equal servings, top with avocado, and serve warm.

Per Serving Calories: 322 | Fat: 22g | Protein: 12g | Sodium: 421mg | Fiber: 8g | Carbohydrates: 19g | Sugar: 8g

Paleo Pancakes

It wouldn't be a cookbook without a classic pancake recipe! You can add your favorite fruit to these pancakes; gently fold it into the batter after mixing. Try serving with warmed maple syrup.

PREP TIME: 10 MINUTES
COOK TIME: 18 MINUTES

INGREDIENTS | SERVES 6

3 large ripe bananas

3 tablespoons cassava flour

2 large eggs

3 tablespoons unsweetened almond milk

½ teaspoon baking soda

½ teaspoon cream of tartar

1. In a medium mixing bowl mash bananas (or use a food processor). Stir in remaining ingredients until well mixed.

2. Heat a griddle pan or skillet over medium heat 3–5 minutes. Using a ¼ measuring cup, pour batter onto griddle and cook until batter bubbles, about 1½–2 minutes. Flip pancake and cook an additional minute. Repeat with remaining batter. Serve warm. Keep in refrigerator up to 3 days.

Per Serving (1 pancake) Calories: 99 | Fat: 2g | Protein: 3g | Sodium: 134mg | Fiber: 2g | Carbohydrates: 19g | Sugar: 8g

Simple Breakfast Bake

This breakfast casserole is easy to throw together when you're having breakfast guests,
or if you want to utilize leftovers for your weekly meal plan.
Try different breakfast meat combinations to keep the dish feeling fresh.

PREP TIME: 20 MINUTES
COOK TIME: 25–35 MINUTES

INGREDIENTS | SERVES 4

¼ cup ghee
1 large white potato, peeled and grated
1 large sweet potato, peeled and grated
1 medium parsnip, peeled and grated
1 small yellow onion, peeled and diced
1 small green bell pepper, seeded and diced
6 large eggs
½ teaspoon fine sea salt
¼ teaspoon ground black pepper
½ pound bacon crumbles
1 cup chopped baby spinach

1. Preheat oven to 350°F. Grease a 9" × 13" baking pan with ghee or coconut oil.

2. In a large skillet over medium-high heat, add ¼ cup ghee, potatoes, parsnip, onion, and bell pepper. Sauté until vegetables are crisp-tender, about 5–7 minutes. Remove from heat.

3. In a medium mixing bowl, stir together remaining ingredients. Add vegetable mixture and stir until well coated. Pour into prepared pan.

4. Bake uncovered 20–30 minutes or until the center passes the toothpick test (if the toothpick comes out clean, the dish is ready). Let stand about 5 minutes before serving. Keep in the refrigerator up to 3 days.

Per Serving   Calories: 651 | Fat: 38g | Protein: 37g | Sodium: 2,355mg | Fiber: 4g | Carbohydrates: 29g | Sugar: 5.5g

Green Disguise

This recipe is a great way to get picky eaters to eat leafy greens in their diet. Because the spinach is chopped, the taste is completely masked by the bacon and eggs. For fans of leafy greens, try doubling the greens in the recipe or leaving them whole.

Egg and Zucchini Scramble

If you're cutting carbs, this recipe is the perfect breakfast for you. Zucchini replaces the presence of starchy potatoes, and a nice helping of healthy fats will keep you feeling full right up until lunch time.

PREP TIME: 10 MINUTES
COOK TIME: 10–15 MINUTES

INGREDIENTS | SERVES 4

¼ cup ghee

1 medium yellow onion, peeled and diced

½ pound ground pork

10 slices bacon, cut into 1" pieces

3 large zucchini, sliced

1 small green bell pepper, seeded and chopped

1 small red bell pepper, seeded and chopped

6 large eggs, beaten

½ teaspoon fine sea salt

½ teaspoon ground black pepper

½ teaspoon onion powder

½ teaspoon garlic powder

¼ teaspoon dried sage

¼ teaspoon dried rosemary

1. In a large skillet over medium heat, add ghee, onion, pork, and bacon and sauté 5–7 minutes or until onion is browned. Add zucchini, green pepper, and red pepper and continue to sauté another 2–3 minutes, stirring frequently.

2. Add remaining ingredients to skillet and stir to mix eggs into other ingredients; cook about 2 minutes, stirring frequently. Remove from heat when eggs are cooked to desired doneness. Serve warm.

Per Serving Calories: 488 | Fat: 34g | Protein: 33g | Sodium: 920mg | Fiber: 2.5g | Carbohydrates: 9.5g | Sugar: 5.5g

Bacon and Parsnip Frittata

You just can't beat the classic flavors of bacon and eggs for breakfast, and this meal swaps parsnips for potatoes, with some added greens for fiber.

PREP TIME: 15 MINUTES
COOK TIME: 30 MINUTES

INGREDIENTS | SERVES 6

3 medium parsnips, peeled and chopped into ½" pieces

4 cups Chicken Stock (see recipe in Chapter 6)

2 tablespoons ghee

1 medium white onion, peeled and chopped

8 slices bacon, cut into 1" pieces

2 cups kale, torn into 1" pieces

8 large eggs, beaten

½ teaspoon fine sea salt

½ teaspoon ground black pepper

½ teaspoon garlic powder

1. Preheat oven to 400°F. In a medium pot over medium heat, boil parsnips in stock until soft, about 15 minutes. Remove from heat and drain.

2. In a medium mixing bowl, stir together remaining ingredients.

3. Spread parsnips evenly on the bottom of a 9" × 13" baking pan and pour egg mixture over top. Bake until eggs are set and the center passes the toothpick test (if the toothpick comes out clean, the dish is ready), about 15 minutes. Remove from oven and let stand 5 minutes before slicing and serving. Keep in refrigerator up to 3 days.

Per Serving   Calories: 284 | Fat: 17g | Protein: 15g | Sodium: 630mg | Fiber: 4g | Carbohydrates: 16g | Sugar: 4.5g

Maple Bacon and Brussels

This breakfast also doubles as the perfect appetizer or side dish, so pop it in the oven when friends are coming over to give your house the sweet, mouthwatering smell of candied bacon.

PREP TIME: 5 MINUTES
COOK TIME: 12–15 MINUTES

INGREDIENTS | SERVES 4

4 cups Brussels sprouts, trimmed and halved

½ cup coconut oil, melted

1 teaspoon sea salt

1 teaspoon onion powder

16 slices bacon

½ cup Grade B maple syrup

1. Preheat oven to 425°F. In a medium mixing bowl stir Brussels sprouts with coconut oil, salt, and onion powder. Spread evenly across a baking sheet. Place bacon strips over Brussels sprouts, covering entire pan. Brush bacon with maple syrup.

2. Bake 12–15 minutes or until bacon is crisp. Be careful not to overcook. Remove from heat and serve warm.

Per Serving   Calories: 524 | Fat: 36g | Protein: 19g | Sodium: 1,381mg | Fiber: 3g | Carbohydrates: 30g | Sugar: 21g

Vegetable Hash with Eggs

You can make this quick-cooking dish with any vegetables you have on hand, and you can easily add any form of meat if you want to make the dish heartier.

PREP TIME: 10 MINUTES
COOK TIME: 15 MINUTES

INGREDIENTS | SERVES 4

2 tablespoons ghee

1 medium yellow onion, peeled and sliced

4 cloves garlic, peeled and chopped

1 large sweet potato, peeled and chopped

1 large turnip, peeled and chopped

1 large white potato, peeled and chopped

½ cup Chicken Stock (see recipe in Chapter 6)

2 cups baby spinach

½ teaspoon fine sea salt

½ teaspoon ground black pepper

½ teaspoon dried thyme

6 large eggs

1. In a large skillet over medium-high heat, cook ghee, onion, garlic, sweet potato, turnip, white potato, and stock until vegetables begin to soften, about 7–10 minutes.

2. Add spinach, seasonings, and eggs and scramble mixture together until eggs are no longer runny and spinach wilts, 4–6 minutes. Serve warm.

Per Serving Calories: 305 | Fat: 15g | Protein: 13.5g | Sodium: 501mg | Fiber: 4g | Carbohydrates: 28.5g | Sugar: 6g

Roasted Vegetables and Eggs

It doesn't get more Paleo than this—a hearty helping of eggs and vegetables. Make this a farmers' market special by using whatever vegetables are in season, and experiment with new combinations!

PREP TIME: 15 MINUTES
COOK TIME: 25–30 MINUTES

INGREDIENTS | SERVES 4

2 heads broccoli, cut into florets
1 cup Brussels sprouts, trimmed and halved
6 medium yellow potatoes, quartered
1 small red onion, peeled and chopped
½ cup ghee
1 teaspoon sea salt
¼ teaspoon ground black pepper
6 large eggs
½ cup bacon crumbles

1. Preheat oven to 425°F. Grease a 9" × 13" baking pan with coconut oil or ghee.

2. In a large mixing bowl stir together broccoli, Brussels sprouts, potatoes, onion, ghee, and seasonings, ensuring vegetables are evenly coated. Spread mixture evenly on the bottom of the baking pan. Bake 10 minutes and then stir vegetables with a wooden spoon, being careful to spread them back out evenly. Bake an additional 5 minutes.

3. Remove pan from oven and reduce heat to 350°F. Crack eggs at even intervals on top of the vegetables, being careful not to break the yolks. Sprinkle bacon crumbles across entire dish. Return pan to oven and bake 10–15 minutes or until whites are not runny and yolks start to solidify. Remove from oven and serve warm.

Per Serving   Calories: 700 | Fat: 41g | Protein: 25g | Sodium: 1,268mg | Fiber: 12g | Carbohydrates: 56.5g | Sugar: 7.5g

CHAPTER 9

Poultry

Slow-Cooked Chicken and Mushrooms

Throw this quick and savory meal in the slow cooker in the morning, and come home to a feast of comfort food and convenience.

PREP TIME: 10 MINUTES
COOK TIME: 4–8 HOURS

INGREDIENTS | SERVES 4

3 pounds boneless, skinless chicken thighs

1 tablespoon ghee

6 cups sliced portobello mushrooms

1 medium yellow onion, peeled and quartered

2 medium carrots, peeled and halved

2 cups Chicken Stock (see recipe in Chapter 6)

3 tablespoons apple cider vinegar

1 teaspoon dried thyme

1 teaspoon garlic powder

1 teaspoon onion powder

½ teaspoon dried basil

½ teaspoon ground black pepper

1 teaspoon coarse Himalayan salt

Add all ingredients to a 6-quart slow cooker, cover, and cook on high 4–5 hours or on low 7–8 hours.

Per Serving Calories: 498 | Fat: 16g | Protein: 70g | Sodium: 1,189mg | Fiber: 4g | Carbohydrates: 13g | Sugar: 6g

Chicken Parts or Whole?

When a recipe calls for chicken thighs, breasts, or wings, you can always substitute what you have on hand, including using a whole bird. This recipe would work just as well with breasts or a whole bird, or even a different kind of white meat such as pork chops or turkey breasts.

Oven-Roasted Chicken and Brussels

This dish will make you rethink Brussels sprouts if you aren't already convinced they're the candy of vegetables. Roasting brings out the sweetness of the Brussels, and the chicken soaks up the apple juice and sea salt, making this the perfect combo of sweet and salty.

PREP TIME: 15 MINUTES
COOK TIME: 30–35 MINUTES

INGREDIENTS | SERVES 4

2 pounds boneless, skinless chicken thighs

2 medium apples, cored and sliced

4 tablespoons avocado oil, divided

2 teaspoons fine sea salt, divided

2 pounds fresh Brussels sprouts, trimmed and halved

½ teaspoon onion powder

1. Preheat oven to 450°F. Line a baking sheet with foil. Place chicken thighs and apples in a 9" × 13" glass baking dish. Drizzle 2 tablespoons avocado oil over chicken and sprinkle with 1 teaspoon salt.

2. In a large mixing bowl, toss sprouts in 1 teaspoon salt, 2 tablespoons oil, and onion powder. Spread evenly on a baking sheet.

3. Place both dishes side by side in oven and bake 15 minutes. Reduce heat to 425°F and continue baking 15–20 minutes or until chicken reaches an internal temperature of 170°F and Brussels sprouts brown and outer leaves crisp up. Remove from oven and serve warm.

Per Serving Calories: 471 | Fat: 19g | Protein: 49g | Sodium: 1,376mg | Fiber: 7g | Carbohydrates: 24g | Sugar: 10g

Balsamic Chicken

This sweet roasted chicken will have you running back for seconds! Pair it with some root vegetables for a meal you won't forget.

PREP TIME: 5 MINUTES
COOK TIME: 20 MINUTES

INGREDIENTS | SERVES 4

2 tablespoons coconut nectar

2 tablespoons balsamic vinegar

½ teaspoon fine sea salt

¼ teaspoon ground black pepper

½ teaspoon onion powder

1 tablespoon avocado oil

4 (6-ounce) boneless, skinless chicken breasts

1. Preheat oven to 400°F. In a small mixing bowl, combine all ingredients except chicken. Whisk together.

2. Evenly space chicken breasts in a 9" × 13" glass baking dish. Brush with coconut nectar mixture and bake 20 minutes or until center of chicken reaches 165°F.

Per Serving Calories: 232 | Fat: 5g | Protein: 36g | Sodium: 232mg | Fiber: 0.1g | Carbohydrates: 6g | Sugar: 6g

Hazelnut Chicken

This recipe calls for hazelnut flour, which brings a nutty twist to breaded chicken. You can make hazelnut flour yourself using a food processor, or you can pick up the Bob's Red Mill brand at your supermarket.

PREP TIME: 10 MINUTES
COOK TIME: 15 MINUTES

INGREDIENTS | SERVES 4

1 large egg, beaten
2 tablespoons ghee
⅔ cup hazelnut flour
⅓ cup almond flour
½ teaspoon fine sea salt
½ teaspoon onion powder
½ teaspoon garlic powder
2 tablespoons avocado oil
4 (6-ounce) boneless, skinless chicken breasts

1. In a small mixing bowl, combine egg and ghee. In a medium mixing bowl, combine hazelnut flour, almond flour, salt, onion powder, and garlic powder.

2. Heat a large skillet over medium-high heat. Add avocado oil. Dip each chicken breast into egg mixture on both sides, and then place in hazelnut mixture until fully coated. Repeat with each breast.

3. Cook breasts in skillet 6–7 minutes per side or until center of chicken reaches 165°F. Serve warm.

Per Serving Calories: 447 | Fat: 28g | Protein: 40g | Sodium: 241mg | Fiber: 2g | Carbohydrates: 5g | Sugar: 0.1g

Apple Honey Mustard Chicken Breasts

This sweet chicken dish is delicious served as whole breasts, or shredded and used for salad toppings or sandwich filling. It's also tasty warm or cold.

PREP TIME: 35 MINUTES
COOK TIME: 35–40 MINUTES

INGREDIENTS | SERVES 4

½ cup unsweetened apple juice
¼ cup apple cider vinegar
¼ cup Sir Kensington's Yellow Mustard
2 tablespoons avocado oil
1 tablespoon coconut sugar
2 tablespoons minced garlic
2 teaspoons coconut aminos
⅛ teaspoon ground black pepper
⅛ teaspoon fine sea salt
4 (6-ounce) boneless, skinless chicken breasts

1. In a small mixing bowl, combine all ingredients except chicken until well mixed.

2. In a large square or rectangular glass baking dish, lay out chicken breasts and pour sauce mixture over them. Turn chicken to coat both sides. Cover and refrigerate 30 minutes.

3. Preheat oven to 350°F. Bake chicken 35–40 minutes or until it reaches an internal temperature of 165°F. Do not overcook. Remove from heat and serve warm.

Per Serving Calories: 295 | Fat: 9g | Protein: 36g | Sodium: 308mg | Fiber: 0.2g | Carbohydrates: 12g | Sugar: 6g

Herbed Chicken, Mushrooms, and Garlic

This dish evokes classic flavors of Grandma's kitchen, and old-fashioned family dinners from simpler days gone by. Serve with roasted potatoes for an updated version of a meat-and-potatoes classic.

PREP TIME: 5 MINUTES
COOK TIME: 4–8 HOURS

INGREDIENTS | SERVES 4

3 pounds skin-on, bone-in chicken breasts and thighs

3 tablespoons ghee

4 cloves garlic, peeled and quartered

1 teaspoon dried basil

1 teaspoon dried rosemary

½ teaspoon dried thyme

½ teaspoon dried sage

½ teaspoon fine Himalayan salt

⅛ teaspoon ground black pepper

½ teaspoon onion powder

1 pound portobello mushrooms, halved

2 cups Chicken Stock (see recipe in Chapter 6)

1 cup water

Add all ingredients to a 6-quart slow cooker, cover, and cook 4–5 hours on high or 7–8 hours on low. Serve warm.

Per Serving   Calories: 533 | Fat: 21g | Protein: 73g | Sodium: 802mg | Fiber: 2g | Carbohydrates: 7g | Sugar: 3g

Savory Chicken and Sweet Potatoes

*This slow cooker dish is the perfect "set it and forget it"
dinner for anyone following the AIP diet—or Paleo in general.*

PREP TIME: 10 MINUTES
COOK TIME: 4–8 HOURS

INGREDIENTS | SERVES 4

2 pounds boneless, skinless chicken thighs

2 large sweet potatoes, peeled and cut into ½" cubes

1 small yellow onion, peeled and quartered

2 tablespoons coconut aminos

2 tablespoons date sugar

2 teaspoons grated ginger

3 cloves garlic, peeled and quartered

1 teaspoon coarse Himalayan salt

3 cups Chicken Stock (see recipe in Chapter 6)

1 cup water

Place all ingredients in a 4-quart slow cooker and stir to combine. Cover and cook on high 4–5 hours or on low 7–8 hours. Serve warm.

Per Serving Calories: 400 | Fat: 10g | Protein: 48g | Sodium: 1,298mg | Fiber: 3g | Carbohydrates: 26.5g | Sugar: 10.5g

Lemon Garlic Chicken Tenders

*These moist chicken cutlets are so tasty that they'll quickly
become the most popular finger food in your house.*

PREP TIME: 5 MINUTES
COOK TIME: 10–15 MINUTES

INGREDIENTS | SERVES 4

2 tablespoons avocado oil

2 pounds chicken tenderloins

2 tablespoons minced garlic

½ teaspoon fine sea salt

¼ teaspoon ground black pepper

2 large lemons, juiced

½ cup Chicken Stock (see recipe in Chapter 6)

1. In a large skillet over medium heat add avocado oil and let warm 2–3 minutes.

2. Add chicken to pan along with remaining ingredients, stirring to combine. Cook 4–6 minutes on each side or until internal temperature of chicken reaches 165°F. Serve warm.

Per Serving Calories: 264 | Fat: 7g | Protein: 45g | Sodium: 652mg | Fiber: 0.3g | Carbohydrates: 3g | Sugar: 0.5g

Spicy Chipotle Pepper Chicken

Use this tasty meat for tacos, salads, or paired with Cauliflower "Rice" (see recipe in Chapter 13), potatoes, or wilted spinach. Cook it ahead of time and use later in the week for quick meals.

PREP TIME: 1 HOUR
COOK TIME: 4–8 HOURS

INGREDIENTS | SERVES 8

8 cloves garlic, peeled and quartered

1 small yellow onion, peeled and quartered

1 small red onion, peeled and quartered

2 tablespoons coconut sugar

1 tablespoon apple cider vinegar

2 tablespoons chili powder

1 teaspoon paprika

1 tablespoon ground cumin

¼ teaspoon red pepper flakes

½ teaspoon fine sea salt

¼ teaspoon ground black pepper

½ teaspoon dried oregano

2 teaspoons onion powder

1 tablespoon Worcestershire sauce

4 cups Chicken Stock (see recipe in Chapter 6)

8 (6-ounce) boneless, skinless chicken breasts

Place all ingredients in a 6-quart slow cooker, cover, and cook 4–5 hours on high or 7–8 hours on low. Let cool about 1 hour, then shred with a fork before serving.

Per Serving   Calories: 248 | Fat: 5g | Protein: 39g | Sodium: 464mg | Fiber: 2g | Carbohydrates: 9g | Sugar: 5g

Roast Turkey and Asparagus

This simple, low-carb dish will leave you satisfied and full without the bloat and discomfort that comes from eating carb-heavy meals.

PREP TIME: 10 MINUTES
COOK TIME: 30–35 MINUTES

INGREDIENTS | SERVES 4

2 pounds turkey breast tenderloins

½ teaspoon onion powder

½ teaspoon garlic powder

2 teaspoons coarse Himalayan salt, divided

½ teaspoon ground black pepper

2 tablespoons avocado oil

32 spears asparagus, ends trimmed

2 tablespoons water

A Rainbow of Asparagus

While green asparagus is what probably comes to mind when you think of this vegetable, it also comes in purple and white varieties. The flavor profile isn't too different among them, although the purple asparagus will have a slightly sweeter taste and the white asparagus will have a slightly blander taste. Any kind or combo will work well for this recipe.

1. Preheat oven to 400°F. In a large glass baking dish, evenly spread out turkey.

2. In a small mixing bowl, combine all seasonings with avocado oil. Spread onto turkey cutlets and place in oven.

3. On a foil-lined baking sheet, spread out asparagus and add water. Cover with tented foil, leaving a slight gap to allow steam to escape. When turkey has been in the oven 10 minutes, place asparagus in oven next to turkey. Continue to cook another 20–25 minutes or until internal temperature of turkey reaches 165°F and asparagus is bright green and tender when speared with a fork. Serve warm.

Per Serving Calories: 342 | Fat: 9g | Protein: 56g | Sodium: 1,018mg | Fiber: 2g | Carbohydrates: 5g | Sugar: 2g

Chicken Onion Stir-Fry

Pair this quick dish with any variety of Paleo "rice" or wrap it in lettuce for a delicious appetizer dish.

PREP TIME: 10 MINUTES
COOK TIME: 15–20 MINUTES

INGREDIENTS | SERVES 4

1 pound boneless, skinless chicken breasts, cut into 1" strips

1 cup Chicken Stock (see recipe in Chapter 6)

3 tablespoons coconut aminos

½ tablespoon apple cider vinegar

1 tablespoon avocado oil

7 green onions, cut into 1" sections

1 cup chopped portobello mushrooms

5 cloves garlic, peeled and sliced

½ teaspoon ground ginger

3 cups snow peas, trimmed

1. In a large skillet or wok over medium-high heat, sauté chicken in stock, aminos, vinegar, and oil about 4–5 minutes, stirring frequently. Add remaining ingredients except snow peas and continue sautéing until chicken is fully cooked, about 8–10 minutes or until the internal temperature reaches 165°F.

2. Add snow peas to skillet and cover with a glass lid, reducing heat to medium. Do not stir. Let snow peas steam on top of mixture 3–5 minutes or until they turn bright green. Remove from heat and serve warm.

Per Serving Calories: 210 | Fat: 6g | Protein: 27g | Sodium: 383mg | Fiber: 2g | Carbohydrates: 9g | Sugar: 3g

Snow Peas Are a Fiber Superfood

While most people will recognize these flat, green pea pods from Asian takeout food, they're actually surprisingly healthy. One cup contains 5 grams of fiber! Cook them lightly for the best flavor, or even enjoy them raw in salads or as a standalone snack.

Spinach Chicken Skillet

This one-dish meal can double as a breakfast if you're looking for a nice break from eggs.

PREP TIME: 5 MINUTES
COOK TIME: 35 MINUTES

INGREDIENTS | SERVES 4

2 medium sweet potatoes, peeled and cubed

3 tablespoons coconut oil

1 teaspoon sea salt

1 tablespoon coconut sugar

3 (6-ounce) boneless, skinless chicken breasts, cubed

1 cup Chicken Stock (see recipe in Chapter 6)

4 cups baby spinach

1. In a large skillet over medium-high heat, sauté sweet potatoes in coconut oil 10 minutes or until potatoes begin to soften. Sprinkle sea salt and coconut sugar in the skillet and stir.

2. Reduce heat to medium and add chicken and stock to skillet. Stirring frequently, cook 20 minutes or until chicken is fully cooked.

3. Add spinach to skillet, stirring well to combine. Cook an additional 5 minutes or until spinach begins to wilt. Remove from heat and serve warm.

Per Serving   Calories: 298 | Fat: 12.5g | Protein: 30g | Sodium: 743mg | Fiber: 2g | Carbohydrates: 14g | Sugar: 6g

Chicken Bok Choy Stir-Fry

Bok choy is one of the lesser-used vegetables in the cruciferous family, but it's just as nutrient rich as broccoli or cabbage. Bok choy is more delicate and produces less of the "gassy" reactions that cruciferous vegetables are often maligned for.

PREP TIME: 5 MINUTES
COOK TIME: 20–30 MINUTES

INGREDIENTS | SERVES 4

2 tablespoons avocado oil

3 (6-ounce) boneless, skinless chicken breasts, cubed

1 cup Chicken Stock (see recipe in Chapter 6)

1 teaspoon fine sea salt

¼ teaspoon finely ground black pepper

½ teaspoon onion powder

½ teaspoon garlic powder

¼ teaspoon ginger powder

½ teaspoon turmeric powder

10 heads baby bok choy, trimmed and sliced

1. In a large skillet or wok over medium heat, warm avocado oil. Add chicken, stock, and seasonings and cook 15–20 minutes or until chicken is fully cooked.

2. Add bok choy to pan and reduce heat to medium-low. Cook an additional 5–10 minutes or until tender. Serve warm.

Per Serving   Calories: 404 | Fat: 11g | Protein: 49g | Sodium: 1,596mg | Fiber: 14.5g | Carbohydrates: 32g | Sugar: 17g

Chicken and Beans

While beans aren't Paleo, green beans are, and this dish pairs versatile chicken with the slight sweetness of fresh green beans, adding in some onion, garlic, and mushrooms to round out the flavors.

PREP TIME: 10 MINUTES
COOK TIME: 25 MINUTES

INGREDIENTS | SERVES 4

3 (6-ounce) boneless, skinless chicken breasts, cubed

1 tablespoon avocado oil

½ teaspoon fine sea salt

1 small yellow onion, peeled and diced

1 tablespoon minced garlic

4 cups water

½ pound portobello mushrooms, sliced

1 pound fresh green beans, trimmed

All about Green Beans

A rich source of vitamin K, green beans are also rich in vitamins A and C, as well as calcium, magnesium, and phosphorus. Additionally, they're an excellent low-carb vegetable choice, and won't spike your blood sugar if you decide to eat a few extra servings.

1. In a large skillet over medium heat, sauté chicken in avocado oil with salt, onion, and garlic until chicken is fully cooked, about 15 minutes. Remove chicken from pan and keep warm. Set aside skillet.

2. In a medium saucepan, heat water until boiling.

3. Meanwhile, sauté mushrooms in the large skillet over high heat until softened, about 3 minutes. Return chicken to pan and continue cooking about 2 minutes.

4. Add green beans in a steamer basket to saucepan, cover, and steam about 5 minutes or until beans turn bright green.

5. Place green beans on plates and top with chicken and mushroom mixture. Serve warm.

Per Serving Calories: 319 | Fat: 6g | Protein: 36g | Sodium: 300mg | Fiber: 10.5g | Carbohydrates: 28.5g | Sugar: 2g

Chicken Apple Patties

These "burgers" can be paired with Paleo bread or served with lettuce wraps for a utensil-free meal. Put down the forks and enjoy these with your hands!

PREP TIME: 15 MINUTES
COOK TIME: 30–35 MINUTES

INGREDIENTS | SERVES 4

1 pound ground chicken

1 small red onion, peeled and diced

1 medium Granny Smith apple, peeled and grated

3 tablespoons cassava flour, plus extra as needed

½ teaspoon fine sea salt

⅛ teaspoon ground black pepper

1. Preheat oven to 350°F. In a small mixing bowl, combine all ingredients using a spoon or your hands. (If mixture looks too wet, add cassava flour 1 teaspoon at a time till desired consistency is achieved.) Make sure everything is thoroughly combined.

2. Line a baking sheet with foil or parchment paper. Separate meat mixture into 4 equal portions and form into patties; space out evenly on baking sheet.

3. Bake patties 30–35 minutes or until center of patty reaches 165°F on a meat thermometer. Remove from oven and serve warm.

Per Serving   Calories: 207 | Fat: 9g | Protein: 20g | Sodium: 348mg | Fiber: 1g | Carbohydrates: 11g | Sugar: 4g

Mango Duck Breast

Slow-cooked mangoes soften and create their own sauce in this easy duck dish.

PREP TIME: 5 MINUTES
COOK TIME: 4 HOURS

INGREDIENTS | SERVES 4

2 boneless, skinless duck breasts

1 large mango, peeled, pitted, and cubed

¼ cup duck or chicken stock

1 tablespoon ginger juice

1 tablespoon minced jalapeño pepper

1 tablespoon minced shallot

Place all ingredients in a 4-quart slow cooker. Cover and cook on low 4 hours.

Per Serving   Calories: 158 | Fat: 3g | Protein: 17.5g | Sodium: 78mg | Fiber: 1.5g | Carbohydrates: 13g | Sugar: 12g

Zesty Chicken and Green Beans

Any green vegetable will work in this skillet dish, so for a change of pace, try broccoli, Broccolini, sugar snap peas, or okra.

PREP TIME: 10 MINUTES
COOK TIME: 15–20 MINUTES

INGREDIENTS | SERVES 4

1 pound fresh green beans, trimmed

4 cups water

1 tablespoon avocado oil

3 (6-ounce) boneless, skinless chicken breasts, cubed

2 tablespoons coconut aminos

1 tablespoon minced garlic

2 teaspoons onion powder

1 teaspoon chili powder

1 large lemon, zested

1 teaspoon raw honey

2 tablespoons whole raw hemp seeds

1. Add green beans to a steamer basket and steam over 4 cups boiling water in a medium saucepan 4–5 minutes or until bright green. Remove from heat and set aside.

2. In a large skillet or wok, heat avocado oil over medium-high heat 1–2 minutes. Add chicken, aminos, spices, lemon zest, and honey. Sauté 5–7 minutes or until chicken is fully cooked, stirring frequently.

3. Add green beans to wok or skillet and cook an additional 2–3 minutes, stirring frequently. Top with raw hemp seeds and serve warm.

Per Serving Calories: 247 | Fat: 7.5g | Protein: 31g | Sodium: 204mg | Fiber: 4g | Carbohydrates: 12.5g | Sugar: 2g

Hemp Nuts?

Hemp seeds, or hemp hearts as they're sometimes referred to, are actually nuts, and an extremely nutritious part of a Paleo diet. They're rich in both omega-6 and omega-3 fatty acids, as well as protein—3 tablespoons provide about 12 grams of protein, making them a great addition for smoothies or quick on-the-go snacking. Toss a handful in your granola after baking it, as cooking neutralizes some of the beneficial fat content of hemp.

Paprika Baked Chicken

This quick and spicy chicken dish can be paired with any starchy vegetable or wrapped in cabbage or lettuce leaves for a tasty finger-food meal.

PREP TIME: 10 MINUTES
COOK TIME: 25 MINUTES

INGREDIENTS | SERVES 4

7 strips bacon, cut into 1" pieces

10 chicken tenderloins, cut into 2" pieces

2 teaspoons fine sea salt

½ teaspoon ground black pepper

2 tablespoons avocado oil

1 large white onion, peeled and sliced

1 large red bell pepper, seeded and sliced into strips

1 large yellow bell pepper, seeded and sliced into strips

1 large green bell pepper, seeded and sliced into strips

1 large zucchini, thinly sliced

2 tablespoons minced garlic

1 teaspoon paprika

1 teaspoon smoked paprika

1 cup Chicken Stock (see recipe in Chapter 6)

2 cups grape tomatoes, halved

1. In a large skillet over medium heat, sauté bacon about 3 minutes. Remove bacon and set aside. Add chicken to pan with bacon drippings along with salt and pepper. Cook about 15 minutes or until chicken is fully cooked (165°F), stirring frequently. Remove chicken from skillet and keep warm.

2. Add remaining ingredients, except tomatoes, to skillet and sauté 5 minutes. Return chicken and bacon to pan, add tomatoes, and cook 2 minutes more. Serve warm.

Per Serving Calories: 375 | Fat: 15g | Protein: 40g | Sodium: 1,807mg | Fiber: 4g | Carbohydrates: 16g | Sugar: 6g

Spiced Chicken

This extra-spicy chicken is the perfect addition to any salad, stir-fry, or lettuce wrap.
Adjust heat level to your personal preference by adding more or less cayenne pepper.

PREP TIME: 35 MINUTES
COOK TIME: 30–35 MINUTES

INGREDIENTS | SERVES 4

2 tablespoons avocado oil

1 small lemon, zested and juiced

1 teaspoon coarse Himalayan salt

½ teaspoon ground black pepper

2 teaspoons ground cumin

½ teaspoon cayenne pepper

½ teaspoon ground cinnamon

½ teaspoon ground coriander

4 (6-ounce) boneless, skinless chicken breasts

1. In a small mixing bowl, combine all ingredients except chicken. Stir well.

2. Spread out chicken on a foil-lined baking sheet. Spread mixture over both sides of chicken. Cover and marinate in refrigerator 30 minutes.

3. Preheat oven to 375°F. Bake chicken 30–35 minutes or until internal temperature reaches 165°F. Serve warm.

Per Serving Calories: 241 | Fat: 8g | Protein: 36g | Sodium: 343mg | Fiber: 1g | Carbohydrates: 2g | Sugar: 0.2g

Chicken Stew with Meat Sauce

This easy-to-make chicken stew is sure to please the entire family.
Both kids and adults love this delicious recipe. Serve alone, over your favorite steamed
vegetable, or over spaghetti squash as a Bolognese-type sauce.

PREP TIME: 5 MINUTES
COOK TIME: 5 HOURS 15 MINUTES

INGREDIENTS | SERVES 4

1 pound (90 percent lean) grassfed ground beef

4 (6-ounce) boneless, skinless chicken breasts, cubed

1 (6-ounce) can tomato paste

1 (28-ounce) can diced tomatoes

4 cloves garlic, peeled and chopped

4 large carrots, peeled and sliced

2 medium red bell peppers, seeded and diced

2 medium green bell peppers, seeded and diced

1 tablespoon dried thyme

2 tablespoons olive oil

1 tablespoon chili powder

1. In a medium sauté pan, cook ground beef until browned, about 5 minutes. Drain and place in a 4-quart slow cooker.

2. Wipe out pan and place over medium-high heat. Brown chicken 5 minutes per side. Add to slow cooker.

3. Combine all remaining ingredients in slow cooker.

4. Cover and cook on high 5 hours.

Per Serving Calories: 512 | Fat: 13g | Protein: 67g | Sodium: 543mg | Fiber: 10g | Carbohydrates: 33g | Sugar: 19g

Slow Cookers Are Lifesavers

Slow cookers are the greatest appliance for the Paleo enthusiast. These little counter-top cookers allow you to cook easily and in bulk, which is important for a successful Paleo diet.

Chopped Chicken Livers

*This chicken liver dish is a perfect appetizer when paired with
Paleo crackers or vegetable sticks, or can serve as the main dish when spread on
Paleo bread or paired with baked eggplant or other root vegetables.*

PREP TIME: 10 MINUTES
COOK TIME: 18–20 MINUTES

INGREDIENTS | SERVES 4

1 pound chicken livers, trimmed
¼ cup olive oil
2 medium onions, peeled and chopped
½ teaspoon ground black pepper
2 large hard-boiled eggs, peeled and chopped

Nutrient-Rich Organ Meats

Organ meat is a great source of protein, vitamin A, and the mineral iron. If chicken liver is not to your liking, you might want to try beef liver, which has more vitamins and minerals and less fat calories per gram.

1. Preheat broiler. Place chicken livers on a baking sheet.

2. Broil chicken livers 8–10 minutes or until cooked thoroughly and no longer pink inside, turning frequently.

3. In a large skillet, heat olive oil over medium heat. Sauté onions 10 minutes or until browned.

4. Place chicken livers, onions, and pepper in a food processor and pulse until coarsely chopped. Pour mixture into a medium bowl.

5. Fold eggs into liver mixture. Serve warm or chilled.

Per Serving Calories: 286 | Fat: 17g | Protein: 23g | Sodium: 113mg | Fiber: 1g | Carbohydrates: 5g | Sugar: 2g

Chicken Enchiladas

If you have been craving a Mexican feast, try this spicy Paleo alternative.
This recipe has most of the taste of traditional enchiladas without the carbohydrates.

PREP TIME: 10 MINUTES
COOK TIME: 25 MINUTES

INGREDIENTS | SERVES 8

2 tablespoons avocado oil

2 pounds boneless, skinless chicken breast, cut into 1" cubes

4 cloves garlic, peeled and minced

½ cup finely chopped onion

2 cups chopped tomatoes

1 teaspoon ground cumin

1 teaspoon chili powder

½ cup chopped fresh cilantro

Juice from 2 large limes

1 (10-ounce) package frozen chopped spinach, thawed and drained

¼ cup sliced green olives

8 collard green leaves

1. Heat oil in a medium frying pan over medium-high heat. Sauté chicken, garlic, and onion in hot oil until thoroughly cooked, about 10 minutes.

2. Add tomatoes, cumin, chili powder, cilantro, and lime juice and simmer 5 minutes.

3. Add spinach and simmer 5 more minutes. Remove from heat. Stir in olives.

4. In a separate medium saucepan, bring 1 cup water to a boil over high heat. Place collard greens in a steamer basket and steam until softened, about 5 minutes.

5. Wrap chicken mixture in collard greens and serve.

Per Serving Calories: 184 | Fat: 5.5g | Protein: 26g | Sodium: 74mg | Fiber: 2g | Carbohydrates: 6g | Sugar: 2g

Turkey Meatballs

This is a fairly generic meatball recipe with some basic additions. You can substitute any type of ground meat you prefer: bison, beef, chicken, or pork. Flaxseed meal can replace the almond meal as well.

PREP TIME: 15 MINUTES
COOK TIME: 20 MINUTES

INGREDIENTS | SERVES 8

2 pounds ground turkey

1 cup almond meal

2 large eggs

5 green onions, chopped

1 medium red bell pepper, seeded and diced

2 cloves garlic, peeled and minced

1 tablespoon dried basil

1 tablespoon dried oregano

2 tablespoons avocado oil

1. Preheat oven to 400°F.

2. Combine all ingredients except oil in a large bowl. Mix well with clean hands.

3. Add oil to turkey mixture and mix well.

4. Form turkey mixture into 24 meatballs and place on 2 baking sheets.

5. Bake 20 minutes.

Per Serving   Calories: 244 | Fat: 1g | Protein: 17g | Sodium: 74mg | Fiber: 2g | Carbohydrates: 4g | Sugar: 0.5g

Fat Content in Ground Meats

Although most people make sure to buy ground meat with the lowest fat content, it is more beneficial to buy fattier ground meat when it is from grassfed or barn-roaming animals. This meat is lower in saturated fat than most commercial ground meat, and the fat profiles favor the omega-3 fatty acids to fight inflammation and heart disease in your body.

Meats

Roasted Steak and Vegetables

The value of this savory dinner is how effortlessly large servings of vegetables are worked in.

PREP TIME: 10 MINUTES
COOK TIME: 30 MINUTES

INGREDIENTS | SERVES 4

2 (8-ounce) sirloin steaks, cut into ½" strips

2 heads broccoli, cut into florets

1 head cauliflower, cut into florets

1 pound Brussels sprouts, trimmed and halved

1 large lemon, juiced

1 teaspoon fine sea salt

½ teaspoon ground black pepper

2 tablespoons avocado oil

2 teaspoons garlic powder

1 teaspoon onion powder

1. Preheat oven to 425°F. In a large skillet over medium-high heat, sear steak until browned, about 2 minutes. Remove from heat and set aside.

2. In a large mixing bowl, toss broccoli, cauliflower, and sprouts with remaining ingredients. Spread on a baking sheet and bake 15 minutes.

3. Add sirloin to baking sheet and cook an additional 10 minutes or until steak reaches desired level of doneness. Vegetables should be browned and starting to crisp. Serve warm.

Per Serving Calories: 479 | Fat: 20g | Protein: 42g | Sodium: 750mg | Fiber: 11g | Carbohydrates: 29g | Sugar: 8g

Mongolian Beef and Broccoli

This Asian-inspired dish will satisfy any cravings you have for takeout, and it's completely Paleo!

PREP TIME: 15 MINUTES
COOK TIME: 3–7 HOURS

INGREDIENTS | SERVES 4

2 pounds beef flank steak, trimmed and cut into ½" strips

1 large white onion, peeled and thinly sliced

½ cup coconut sugar

½ cup coconut aminos

2 tablespoons Worcestershire sauce

4½ cups water, divided

1 tablespoon gelatin

2 tablespoons minced garlic

2 heads broccoli, cut into florets

3 green onions, sliced

1. Add all ingredients except 4 cups water, broccoli, and green onions to a 6-quart slow cooker. Cover and cook on high 3–4 hours or on low 6–7 hours.

2. About 15 minutes before serving, steam broccoli 3–4 minutes in a steamer basket over 4 cups boiling water in a medium saucepan until bright green. Do not overcook.

3. Top with beef, garnish with green onions, and serve warm.

Per Serving Calories: 538 | Fat: 12g | Protein: 55g | Sodium: 950mg | Fiber: 5g | Carbohydrates: 47.5g | Sugar: 29.5g

Paleo Mushu Pork

The sweetness of the coconut aminos plays nicely with the pungent onions and salty Asian-inspired flavors of this paleoized dish, which pairs perfectly with Jicama "Rice" (see recipe in Chapter 13).

PREP TIME: 10 MINUTES
COOK TIME: 10–15 MINUTES

INGREDIENTS | SERVES 4

2 tablespoons avocado oil

4 (4-ounce) boneless pork chops, cut into ½" strips

8 ounces white button mushrooms, sliced

6 green onions, sliced

1 medium head green cabbage, shredded

2 large carrots, peeled and shredded

3 tablespoons coconut aminos

⅛ teaspoon red pepper flakes

½ teaspoon fine sea salt

1. In a wok or large skillet over medium-high heat, heat avocado oil until it just starts to bubble. Add pork strips and sauté 3–4 minutes or until center is just a little pink. Remove from heat and set aside.

2. Add remaining ingredients to wok or skillet and sauté 4–5 minutes or until mushrooms are softened and cabbage is wilted. Stir frequently. Add pork back to pan and cook 1–2 minutes more. Serve warm.

Per Serving Calories: 280 | Fat: 10g | Protein: 28g | Sodium: 910mg | Fiber: 6g | Carbohydrates: 18g | Sugar: 3g

Cinnamon Pork Chops and Pears

This easy slow-cooker dish evokes warm flavors that pair perfectly with roasted root vegetables such as beets, turnips, and sweet potatoes.

PREP TIME: 5 MINUTES
COOK TIME: 3–6 HOURS

INGREDIENTS | SERVES 4

4 (8-ounce) boneless pork chops

½ tablespoon ground cinnamon

2 tablespoons coconut sugar

½ teaspoon fine sea salt

4 Anjou pears, cored and sliced

1 cup water

Place all ingredients in a 6-quart slow cooker. Use a wooden spoon to swirl seasonings into water, evenly coating pears and pork chops. Add more water if necessary so the chops are just covered by liquid. Cover and cook 3–4 hours on high or 5–6 hours on low. Serve warm.

Per Serving Calories: 352 | Fat: 6g | Protein: 48g | Sodium: 913mg | Fiber: 3g | Carbohydrates: 22g | Sugar: 16g

Roast Beef and Baby Potatoes

*This recipe will fill you up, and to get some greens on your plate,
it pairs nicely with steamed green beans.*

PREP TIME: 20 MINUTES
COOK TIME: 4–11 HOURS

INGREDIENTS | SERVES 4

1 (3-pound) beef roast

2 pounds small red potatoes, halved

1 large yellow onion, peeled and quartered

4 large carrots, peeled and cut into 1" sections

3 tablespoons minced garlic

1 tablespoon onion powder

2 teaspoons fine sea salt

1 teaspoon ground black pepper

1. In a large skillet over high heat, sear beef roast on all sides until browned. Remove from heat and add to a 6-quart slow cooker.

2. Add remaining ingredients to slow cooker. Cover and cook on high heat 4–5 hours or on low heat 7–8 hours. For an extra-tender roast, remove potatoes and continue to cook roast on low heat an additional 2–3 hours. Serve warm.

Per Serving   Calories: 733 | Fat: 19.5g | Protein: 80g | Sodium: 1,363mg | Fiber: 7g | Carbohydrates: 50g | Sugar: 8g

Asian Bison and Noodle Bowl

This twist on a takeout dish will have diners doing a double-take—the bison is a leaner version of red meat, and the kelp noodles are the perfect gluten-free, Paleo-friendly substitute for rice noodles.

PREP TIME: 5 MINUTES
COOK TIME: 40–45 MINUTES

INGREDIENTS | SERVES 4

2 (8-ounce) bison steaks, cubed

3 tablespoons avocado oil

4 cups Beef Stock (see recipe in Chapter 6)

1 small yellow onion, peeled and finely sliced

3 tablespoons coconut aminos

1 tablespoon fish sauce

2 tablespoons minced garlic

16 ounces kelp noodles

In a large skillet or wok, cook bison in avocado oil over medium heat 5 minutes. Add remaining ingredients and reduce heat to medium-low. Simmer 35–40 minutes or until noodles are softened, stirring occasionally. Serve warm.

Per Serving   Calories: 348 | Fat: 19g | Protein: 30g | Sodium: 1,256mg | Fiber: 2g | Carbohydrates: 11g | Sugar: 2g

Broccoli and Pancetta Stir-Fry

The salty pancetta combines with the slightly bitter broccoli flavor to create a perfectly savory combo that pairs well with Jicama "Rice" (see recipe in Chapter 13) or wrapped in large cabbage leaves.

PREP TIME: 15 MINUTES
COOK TIME: 15 MINUTES

INGREDIENTS | SERVES 4

2 large heads broccoli, florets and stems separated

1 pound pancetta, cut into 1" pieces

¼ cup coconut aminos

1 tablespoon coconut sugar

⅛ teaspoon red pepper flakes

1 tablespoon minced garlic

1 tablespoon onion powder

1. Using a spiralizer or a grater, spiralize or grate broccoli stems. Alternately, use a food processor to cut them into matchsticks.

2. In a large skillet or wok over medium-high heat, cook pancetta for 5–7 minutes, stirring frequently. Add broccoli stems and florets along with remaining ingredients. Sauté 5–7 minutes or until broccoli starts to soften, stirring frequently. Serve warm or chilled.

Per Serving Calories: 626 | Fat: 45g | Protein: 25g | Sodium: 1,708mg | Fiber: 8g | Carbohydrates: 33g | Sugar: 8.5g

Sausage and Potatoes

This spicy one-pan dish can easily double as a breakfast or a high-protein snack. Pair it with some greens for a well-rounded diet.

PREP TIME: 10 MINUTES
COOK TIME: 30 MINUTES

INGREDIENTS | SERVES 4

1 pound ground pork sausage

1 tablespoon ghee

2 medium sweet potatoes, peeled and cubed

2 tablespoons coconut oil

½ teaspoon fine sea salt

¼ teaspoon ground black pepper

¼ teaspoon onion powder

1 large ripe avocado, peeled and sliced

1. In a large skillet over medium heat, cook sausage in ghee until browned, about 10 minutes. Remove from skillet and set aside.

2. In the same skillet, add potatoes, oil, and seasonings. Cook potatoes until soft, about 20 minutes. Stir often to cook evenly.

3. Stir sausage back into skillet with potatoes. Spoon into serving bowls, top with avocado slices, and serve immediately.

Per Serving Calories: 327 | Fat: 19g | Protein: 25.5g | Sodium: 385mg | Fiber: 4g | Carbohydrates: 13g | Sugar: 3g

Hawaiian Stir-Fry

This sweet and spicy stir-fry dish tastes like summer on a plate!

PREP TIME: 2 HOURS
COOK TIME: 10 MINUTES

INGREDIENTS | SERVES 4

¼ cup coconut aminos

2 teaspoons avocado oil

1 tablespoon raw honey

1 teaspoon lemon juice

1 teaspoon apple cider vinegar

1 teaspoon Worcestershire sauce

2 (8-ounce) sirloin steaks, cut into 1" strips

2 tablespoons coconut oil

2 tablespoons minced garlic

1 large green bell pepper, seeded and cut into strips

1 large yellow bell pepper, seeded and cut into strips

2 teaspoons coconut nectar

1 teaspoon coarse Himalayan salt

1 cup cubed pineapple

3 clementines, peeled and separated

1. In a medium mixing bowl, whisk together coconut aminos, avocado oil, honey, lemon juice, vinegar, and Worcestershire.

2. In a medium glass dish, lay out sirloin strips and cover with marinade. Cover and refrigerate 1½–2 hours.

3. In a wok or large skillet over medium-high heat, heat coconut oil until bubbling, about 2 minutes. Add marinated steak and stir-fry 2–3 minutes. Remove steak from wok, leaving marinade behind. Add remaining ingredients and stir-fry 3–5 minutes, stirring frequently. Return beef to wok, cook 1 minute more, and serve warm.

Per Serving Calories: 482 | Fat: 25g | Protein: 32g | Sodium: 714mg | Fiber: 2g | Carbohydrates: 25g | Sugar: 15g

Balsamic Steak Sauté

Any red meat will work for this dish, so try using different cuts of steak, or other red meats, such as lamb or buffalo. Wrap in lettuce or serve with roasted Brussels sprouts for a delicious, low-carb meal.

PREP TIME: 2 HOURS
COOK TIME: 8 MINUTES

INGREDIENTS | SERVES 4

3 (6-ounce) sirloin steaks, cut into 1" strips

½ cup balsamic vinegar

2 tablespoons avocado oil

2 tablespoons raw honey

½ teaspoon fine sea salt

¼ teaspoon ground black pepper

¼ teaspoon onion powder

1. Place steak strips in a medium glass bowl. In a small mixing bowl, whisk together vinegar, oil, honey, and seasonings. Pour over steak strips. Cover and marinate in refrigerator 1½–2 hours.

2. Preheat a large skillet over medium-high heat 3 minutes. Add steak strips and sauté–about 5 minutes or until steak reaches preferred level of doneness, stirring frequently. Let rest 5 minutes before serving warm.

Per Serving Calories: 405 | Fat: 20g | Protein: 36g | Sodium: 301mg | Fiber: 0.1g | Carbohydrates: 11g | Sugar: 10g

Lamb Burgers

This twist on an American classic freshens up the notion of a burger, and when paired with large lettuce leaves, onions, and tomatoes, this dish will quickly become part of your regular rotation.

PREP TIME: 10 MINUTES
COOK TIME: 15 MINUTES

INGREDIENTS | SERVES 4

1 pound ground lamb

1 large egg

2 teaspoons garlic powder

1 teaspoon onion powder

½ teaspoon fine sea salt

¼ teaspoon ground black pepper

5 green onions, sliced

2 medium Roma tomatoes, sliced

4 large leaves romaine lettuce

1. In a medium mixing bowl, combine lamb, egg, seasonings, and onions until thoroughly mixed. Flatten into 4 equal patties.

2. Preheat a large skillet or grill pan on medium heat 3 minutes. Add burgers and cook on one side 6–7 minutes; turn and cook an additional 5–6 minutes for medium. Adjust cooking times for preferred level of doneness.

3. Remove from heat and let rest 5 minutes. Top with tomato slices and wrap in lettuce. Serve warm.

Per Serving Calories: 368 | Fat: 26g | Protein: 22g | Sodium: 371mg | Fiber: 1.5g | Carbohydrates: 7g | Sugar: 4g

Ginger Shredded Pork

This slow-cooker meal will be the answer to "what's for dinner?" every day of the week once you've tasted this sweet and hot, melt-in-your-mouth pork. Serve with Jicama "Rice" (see recipe in Chapter 13) or roasted potatoes.

PREP TIME: 10 MINUTES
COOK TIME: 4–8 HOURS

INGREDIENTS | SERVES 4

4 (6-ounce) boneless pork chops
2 large oranges, juiced
1 small lemon, juiced
2 tablespoons coconut aminos
2 teaspoons sesame oil
1 tablespoon ground ginger
1 teaspoon fine sea salt
¼ teaspoon ground black pepper
2 teaspoons garlic powder
2 teaspoons onion powder
2 tablespoons blackstrap molasses

Add all ingredients to a 6-quart slow cooker, cover, and cook on high heat 4–5 hours or on low heat 7–8 hours. Shred meat with a fork and serve warm.

Per Serving Calories: 304 | Fat: 7g | Protein: 37g | Sodium: 1,208mg | Fiber: 1g | Carbohydrates: 20g | Sugar: 13g

Paleo Spaghetti Carbonara

This paleoized version of the classic Italian dish makes up for its lack of cheese by offering a rich, buttery sauce.

PREP TIME: 15 MINUTES
COOK TIME: 10 MINUTES

INGREDIENTS | SERVES 4

6 ounces pancetta, finely chopped
2 large eggs
½ teaspoon ground black pepper
½ teaspoon fine sea salt
1 cup ghee
5 large zucchini, spiralized
2 cups coarsely chopped kale
2 cups baby spinach

1. In a large skillet over medium-high heat, sauté pancetta 3 minutes or until browned. Remove pancetta from skillet and set aside.

2. In a medium mixing bowl, whisk together eggs, seasonings, and ghee.

3. Add zucchini to skillet over medium heat and cover with egg mixture. Stir continuously, until zucchini begins to soften, about 3 minutes. Add kale and spinach and cook an additional 2–3 minutes until leaves begin to wilt. Remove from heat, top with pancetta, and serve immediately.

Per Serving Calories: 809 | Fat: 80g | Protein: 13g | Sodium: 825mg | Fiber: 3g | Carbohydrates: 11g | Sugar: 6.5g

Eggplant Steaks

Eggplant has to be salted before it is cooked or it will release too much moisture and will steam instead of grilling. Topping the eggplant with a sauce made from sun-dried tomatoes makes this a very appealing meal.

PREP TIME: 1 HOUR 30 MINUTES
COOK TIME: 6–8 MINUTES

INGREDIENTS | SERVES 4

2 large eggplant, cut into ¾"-thick slices

1 tablespoon plus ¼ teaspoon sea salt, divided

1 cup hot water

6 sun-dried tomatoes (not packed in oil)

¼ cup plus 3 tablespoons olive oil, divided

⅓ cup almond meal

1 tablespoon lemon juice

2 teaspoons fresh thyme leaves

⅛ teaspoon ground white pepper

1. Place eggplant slices on a baking sheet and sprinkle with 1 tablespoon salt. Let stand 1 hour.

2. Rinse eggplant thoroughly under cool running water. Place between paper towels and press down to remove moisture.

3. Combine hot water and sun-dried tomatoes in a small bowl; let stand 15 minutes to rehydrate. Remove tomatoes from water and coarsely chop.

4. In food processor or blender, combine ¼ cup oil, tomatoes, almond meal, lemon juice, thyme, ¼ teaspoon salt, and pepper. Blend until combined.

5. Prepare and preheat grill on medium. Brush eggplant with 3 tablespoons olive oil and place on grill rack. Grill 6–8 minutes, turning once, until eggplant slices are tender with nice grill marks. Top each with a spoonful of tomato mixture and serve immediately.

Per Serving Calories: 319 | Fat: 27g | Protein: 3g | Sodium: 1,552mg | Fiber: 8g | Carbohydrates: 17g | Sugar: 9g

Roasted Pork Tenderloin

When you are preparing for a large family gathering and find yourself with a bit more time than expected, this is the recipe to go for. It serves 10 easily and will wow your guests with its flavorful punch.

PREP TIME: 2 HOURS 45 MINUTES
COOK TIME: 20–25 MINUTES

INGREDIENTS | SERVES 10

1 (2½-pound) pork loin
Juice of 1 large orange
3 tablespoons lime juice
2 tablespoons red wine
10 cloves garlic, peeled and minced
2 tablespoons dried rosemary
1 tablespoon ground black pepper

1. Combine all ingredients in a shallow dish or large zip-top plastic bag. Refrigerate and marinate pork at least 2 hours or up to overnight.

2. Remove pork from marinade and bring to room temperature. Preheat oven to 350°F.

3. In a roasting pan, cook uncovered 20–25 minutes or until internal temperature reaches 165°F. Allow pork to rest 5 minutes before carving.

Per Serving   Calories: 186 | Fat: 9g | Protein: 23.5g | Sodium: 73mg | Fiber: 0.5g | Carbohydrates: 3g | Sugar: 0.3g

Grassfed Lamb Meatballs

Meatballs are always a kid favorite. These grassfed lamb meatballs are high in good fats that contribute to their great taste and nutrition.

PREP TIME: 15 MINUTES
COOK TIME: 15 MINUTES

INGREDIENTS | SERVES 6

¼ cup pine nuts
4 tablespoons olive oil, divided
1½ pounds ground grassfed lamb
¼ cup minced garlic
2 tablespoons ground cumin

1. Over medium-high heat sauté pine nuts in 2 tablespoons olive oil about 2 minutes until browned. Remove from pan and let cool.

2. In a large bowl, combine lamb, garlic, cumin, and pine nuts and form into 1½" meatballs.

3. Add remaining olive oil to pan and fry meatballs until cooked through, about 5–7 minutes.

Per Serving   Calories: 416 | Fat: 32g | Protein: 28g | Sodium: 91mg | Fiber: 0.5g | Carbohydrates: 3.5g | Sugar: 0.3g

Beef Brisket with Onions and Mushrooms

This recipe makes a roast so packed with flavor it will melt in your mouth.

PREP TIME: 35 MINUTES
COOK TIME: 4 HOURS

INGREDIENTS | SERVES 4

4 cloves garlic, peeled

1½ teaspoons sea salt, divided

4 tablespoons avocado oil, divided

2 teaspoons chopped fresh rosemary

1 (1-pound) beef brisket

1 teaspoon ground black pepper

3 large onions, peeled and quartered

3 cups sliced white mushrooms

3 medium stalks celery, cut into large chunks

2 cups Beef Stock (see recipe in Chapter 6)

1 (16-ounce) can whole tomatoes, chopped

2 bay leaves

Kitchen Gadgets

The mortar and pestle was originally used in pharmacies to crush ingredients together to make medicines. In the culinary world, the mortar and pestle is a very useful tool for crushing seeds and nuts and making guacamole, pesto, and garlic paste.

1. Preheat oven to 325°F.

2. Using a mortar and pestle or the back of a spoon and a small bowl, mash together garlic, ½ teaspoon salt, 2 tablespoons oil, and rosemary to make a paste.

3. Season brisket with pepper and 1 teaspoon salt.

4. Heat remaining oil in a large frying pan and sear brisket over medium-high heat to make a dark crust on both sides. Place in a large roasting pan and spread rosemary paste on brisket. Place onions, mushrooms, and celery in the pan around brisket. Pour stock and tomatoes over brisket and add bay leaves.

5. Tightly cover pan with foil and place in oven. Bake about 4 hours, basting with pan juices every 30 minutes, until beef is very tender.

6. Let brisket rest 15 minutes before slicing it across the grain at a slight diagonal. Remove bay leaves before serving.

Per Serving Calories: 528 | Fat: 36g | Protein: 26.5g | Sodium: 1,248mg | Fiber: 4.5g | Carbohydrates: 18g | Sugar: 8g

Rosemary Rack of Lamb in Berries Sauce

This rack of lamb recipe is sure to be a winner at any holiday or dinner party.
The flavors are strong and the presentation is sure to please.

PREP TIME: 15 MINUTES
COOK TIME: 23 MINUTES

INGREDIENTS | SERVES 4

1 rack grassfed lamb on the bone (about 1 pound)

1 teaspoon ground black pepper

2 cloves garlic, peeled and crushed, divided

1½ teaspoons dried thyme

2 sprigs fresh rosemary, divided

2 tablespoons olive oil

1 cup mixed berries

1 cup Beef Stock (see recipe in Chapter 6)

1. Preheat oven to 400°F.

2. Place rack of lamb in a roasting pan with a rack. Sprinkle lamb with pepper, 1 clove garlic, thyme, and 1 sprig rosemary.

3. Roast 13 minutes per pound or until internal temperature reaches 135°F for medium, 145°F for medium-well, or 155°F for well-done. Remove from oven and set aside to rest.

4. Prepare sauce by combining remaining garlic, remaining rosemary, oil, berries, and stock in a medium saucepan over low heat. Stir and cook about 10 minutes or until mixture reduces and thickens.

5. Pour sauce over lamb and serve warm.

Per Serving Calories: 471 | Fat: 39g | Protein: 18g | Sodium: 74mg | Fiber: 2g | Carbohydrates: 6g | Sugar: 2g

Paleo Meatballs and Sauce

These meatballs are so close to traditional meatballs, you won't know the difference.

PREP TIME: 15 MINUTES
COOK TIME: 4–8 HOURS

INGREDIENTS | SERVES 6

1 (16-ounce) can diced tomatoes

1 (4-ounce) can tomato paste

2 pounds grassfed ground beef

1 cup chopped celery

1 cup peeled and chopped onion

1 cup peeled and chopped carrots

4 cloves garlic, peeled and finely chopped

3 large eggs

½ cup almond flour

1 tablespoon dried oregano

1 teaspoon ground black pepper

¼ teaspoon chili powder

1. Pour canned tomatoes and tomato paste into 4- or 6-quart slow cooker.

2. Place all remaining ingredients in a large bowl and mix well with clean hands.

3. Roll meat mixture into large, rounded tablespoon-sized balls and add to slow cooker.

4. Cover and cook on high 4–5 hours or low 6–8 hours.

Per Serving   Calories: 313 | Fat: 10g | Protein: 39g | Sodium: 208mg | Fiber: 5g | Carbohydrates: 16g | Sugar: 7g

CHAPTER 11

Fish and Seafood

Citrus-Cooked Scallops with Spinach

*The citrus fruit adds mouthwatering flavor to the melt-in-your-mouth scallops,
making this a crowd-pleasing meal for any day of the week.*

PREP TIME: 5 MINUTES
COOK TIME: 6–7 MINUTES

INGREDIENTS | SERVES 4

6 cups baby spinach

1 large red grapefruit, peeled and separated

1 large navel orange, peeled and separated

2 clementines, peeled and separated

1 tablespoon coconut oil at room temperature

½ teaspoon fine sea salt

¼ teaspoon ground black pepper

2 pounds large scallops

1. Place spinach in a large glass bowl. Set aside.

2. In a large skillet over medium-high heat, sauté fruit in coconut oil with salt and pepper 2–3 minutes. Add fruit to spinach, reserving juices in pan.

3. Add scallops to pan and sauté 2 minutes each side or until golden brown. Place on top of spinach, drizzling remaining juices from pan over spinach for the dressing. Serve immediately.

Per Serving Calories: 291 | Fat: 4g | Protein: 30.5g | Sodium: 1,204mg | Fiber: 5g | Carbohydrates: 32g | Sugar: 19.5g

Teriyaki-Glazed Salmon

*Pair this salmon with Cauliflower "Rice" (see recipe in Chapter 13)
or roasted vegetables for a sweet and savory dish that is quick to prepare.*

PREP TIME: 35 MINUTES
COOK TIME: 12–15 MINUTES

INGREDIENTS | SERVES 4

4 (6-ounce) skin-on salmon fillets, thawed or fresh

¼ cup coconut aminos

1 tablespoon Grade B maple syrup

½ tablespoon apple cider vinegar

½ teaspoon ground ginger

½ teaspoon garlic powder

½ teaspoon onion powder

⅛ teaspoon ground black pepper

½ teaspoon fine sea salt

1. In a large glass baking dish, lay salmon fillets skin side down. In a small mixing bowl, whisk together remaining ingredients. Pour over salmon and cover. Refrigerate 30 minutes.

2. Preheat oven to 375°F. Place marinated salmon in baking dish in oven and bake 12–15 minutes or until center of salmon flakes easily. Serve warm.

Per Serving Calories: 275 | Fat: 10g | Protein: 23g | Sodium: 694mg | Fiber: 0.1g | Carbohydrates: 7g | Sugar: 3g

Simple Baked Halibut

Not sure what to make for dinner?
Skip lengthy prep by throwing this fish into the oven for a quick, healthy meal.

PREP TIME: 5 MINUTES
COOK TIME: 10–20 MINUTES

INGREDIENTS | SERVES 4

4 (4-ounce) halibut fillets, fresh or frozen
2 tablespoons ghee
2 tablespoons avocado oil
1 teaspoon paprika
½ cup lemon juice

1. Preheat oven to 400°F. Line a baking sheet with foil, and place halibut fillets skin side down (if they have skin).

2. Using a basting brush, brush fillets first with ghee, then with oil. Sprinkle with paprika. Pour lemon juice onto baking sheet so that the fish can absorb it as it cooks.

3. Bake 10–12 minutes if thawed, 17–20 minutes if frozen. Fully cooked fish should flake easily apart with a fork. Serve warm.

Per Serving Calories: 206 | Fat: 12g | Protein: 21g | Sodium: 77mg | Fiber: 0.3g | Carbohydrates: 2g | Sugar: 1g

Peppery Sautéed Tuna Steaks

A nice alternative to red-meat steaks, tuna steaks have a similar texture
but a much milder flavor that pairs well with a peppery spice blend.

PREP TIME: 5 MINUTES
COOK TIME: 10–12 MINUTES

INGREDIENTS | SERVES 4

¼ cup ghee
4 (6-ounce) tuna steaks
2 tablespoons lemon juice
1 tablespoon avocado oil
½ teaspoon fine sea salt
½ teaspoon ground black pepper
⅛ teaspoon chili pepper

In a large skillet over medium-high heat, warm ghee until it bubbles, about 2 minutes. Add tuna, lemon juice, oil, salt, black pepper, and chili pepper. Cook tuna 4–5 minutes each side, and serve warm.

Per Serving Calories: 381 | Fat: 22g | Protein: 40g | Sodium: 346mg | Fiber: 0.1g | Carbohydrates: 1g | Sugar: 0.2g

Baked Cod with Olives

The simplicity of this dish is deceptive—the flavors will taste like you spent hours preparing it!
Pair it with a slaw (see Chapter 12) for a fresh plate that will rival that of any seaside restaurant.

PREP TIME: 5 MINUTES
COOK TIME: 15 MINUTES

INGREDIENTS | SERVES 4

4 (6-ounce) cod fillets, thawed or fresh
½ teaspoon fine sea salt
¼ teaspoon ground black pepper
2 tablespoons extra-virgin olive oil
2 tablespoons avocado oil
2 tablespoons lemon juice
2 tablespoons minced garlic
½ cup black olives, pitted
¼ cup whole raw hemp seeds

Fish for Fish

Any whitefish will work with this recipe, and
even salmon will too, but it may need to be
cooked slightly longer. Change up the flavors by swapping lime for lemon juice, chili
powder for black pepper, and even try
throwing in some raw honey for a sweet
and spicy spin.

1. Preheat oven to 400°F. Lay fish fillets in a large glass
   baking dish or on a foil-lined baking sheet.

2. In a small mixing bowl, stir together salt, pepper, oils,
   lemon juice, and garlic. Brush over fish, setting aside
   extra.

3. Bake 10–12 minutes or until fish flakes easily with a
   fork.

4. Meanwhile, in a medium skillet over medium heat, add
   remaining oil mixture and sauté olives 2–4 minutes.
   Place on top of fish fillets before serving, and top with
   raw hemp seeds.

Per Serving Calories: 348 | Fat: 20g | Protein: 34g | Sodium:
495mg | Fiber: 1g | Carbohydrates: 4g | Sugar: 0.2g

Shrimp Curry with Pineapple Relish

The "sugar and spice" flavorings of this dish pair nicely with Jicama "Rice" or Cauliflower "Rice" (see Chapter 13). Make the dish ahead of time for easy packable lunches or a quick reheatable dinner for busy evenings.

PREP TIME: 15 MINUTES
COOK TIME: 20–25 MINUTES

INGREDIENTS | SERVES 4

1 small pineapple, peeled, cored, and finely chopped

3 green onions, sliced

1 small lime, juiced

1 small lemon, juiced

2 clementines, peeled and separated

⅛ teaspoon cayenne pepper

1 teaspoon fine sea salt, divided

2 tablespoons ghee

2 pounds fresh or thawed medium shrimp, peeled and deveined

1 tablespoon minced garlic

2 teaspoons onion powder

1 tablespoon turmeric powder

2 teaspoons ground cinnamon

1 teaspoon ground ginger

8 ounces full-fat coconut milk

1. In a small glass bowl, stir together pineapple, onions, lime and lemon juice, clementines, cayenne, and ½ teaspoon sea salt. Refrigerate until needed.

2. In a large skillet over medium heat, warm ghee until it bubbles, about 2 minutes; sauté shrimp 3 minutes. Remove shrimp from pan and set aside.

3. Add remaining ingredients to the same pan. Bring mixture to a boil, then reduce heat to medium-low and simmer 12 minutes.

4. Add shrimp to coconut milk mixture and continue simmering an additional 3–5 minutes or until shrimp is bright pink and no longer looks translucent. Serve topped with pineapple relish.

Per Serving   Calories: 444 | Fat: 21g | Protein: 34g | Sodium: 1,854mg | Fiber: 4g | Carbohydrates: 30g | Sugar: 16g

Can't Stand the Heat?

Reduce the spice of this dish by leaving out the cayenne pepper and halving the turmeric, cinnamon, and ginger. This will make the flavor milder for anyone who is less tolerant of spicy foods, including children.

Baked Mahi-Mahi

This simple fish dish works with any variety of whitefish,
as well as chicken or turkey (however, cooking times will be longer for poultry).

PREP TIME: 5 MINUTES
COOK TIME: 10–12 MINUTES

INGREDIENTS | SERVES 4

4 (6-ounce) mahi-mahi fillets, thawed
2 large lemons, zested and juiced
2 tablespoons avocado oil
1 large lime, zested and juiced
1 teaspoon coarse Himalayan salt
¼ teaspoon ground black pepper
¼ cup ghee

1. Preheat oven to 400°F. Lay fish fillets in a large glass baking dish.

2. In a small mixing bowl, whisk together remaining ingredients and brush over fish fillets, pouring extra in the pan. Bake 10–12 minutes or until center of fish flakes easily with a fork. Serve warm.

Per Serving Calories: 306 | Fat: 19g | Protein: 30g | Sodium: 445mg | Fiber: 1g | Carbohydrates: 2g | Sugar: 0.5g

Thai Coconut Scallops

These scallops cook in 15 minutes and taste as if you were cooking all day.
Great for dinner or for special occasions.

PREP TIME: 5 MINUTES
COOK TIME: 15 MINUTES

INGREDIENTS | SERVES 4

1 tablespoon olive oil
1 pound large scallops
½ medium onion, peeled and chopped
1 (13.66-ounce) can full-fat coconut milk
2 tablespoons hot curry powder
1 teaspoon ground cumin
¼ cup unsweetened coconut flakes
8–10 leaves fresh basil, slivered

1. Heat olive oil in a medium skillet over medium-high heat. Add scallops and onion and sauté until scallops are golden brown, about 2 minutes on each side.

2. Add coconut milk, curry powder, cumin, and coconut flakes. Bring to a light boil and simmer 10 minutes.

3. Garnish with basil.

Per Serving Calories: 346 | Fat: 26g | Protein: 17g | Sodium: 461mg | Fiber: 3g | Carbohydrates: 11g | Sugar: 1g

Salmon Cakes

These salmon cakes are a great party appetizer.
Even non-Paleo dieters will rave about them.

PREP TIME: 10 MINUTES
COOK TIME: 8 MINUTES

INGREDIENTS | SERVES 10

3 pounds salmon, finely diced
5 large egg whites
1 teaspoon dried dill
¼ teaspoon ground ginger
¼ teaspoon cayenne pepper
¼ cup ground black pepper
¼ cup freshly squeezed lemon juice
¼ cup sesame oil
2 tablespoons arrowroot powder
1 cup almond meal

1. Preheat broiler.

2. Mix together all ingredients except almond meal in a large bowl.

3. Form about 20 small patties from mixture.

4. Pour almond meal into a shallow dish. Dredge patties in almond meal and place on an ungreased baking sheet.

5. Broil on each side 4 minutes. Serve warm.

Per Serving Calories: 301 | Fat: 16g | Protein: 29g | Sodium: 87mg | Fiber: 1g | Carbohydrates: 4g | Sugar: 0.3g

Super Omega

The more omega-3 fatty acid you ingest, the better chance you will have at fighting silent inflammation. It is also proven to significantly reduce your recovery time from workouts or endurance races. The more omega-3, the better for optimum health all around.

CHAPTER 12

Salads

Shrimp and Chard Salad

This savory salad dish is easily prepped a day ahead for a quick meal-on-the-go or a packable lunch.

PREP TIME: 10 MINUTES
COOK TIME: 12 MINUTES

INGREDIENTS | SERVES 2

4 slices bacon

12 raw medium shrimp, peeled and deveined

½ cup water

2 tablespoons avocado oil

1 tablespoon lemon juice

¼ teaspoon fine sea salt

¼ teaspoon ground black pepper

2 cups roughly chopped Swiss chard

1 cup arugula

1 cup roughly chopped romaine lettuce

2 cups baby spinach

2 medium Roma tomatoes, sliced

2 large eggs, hard-boiled and peeled

Boiling Eggs

To make your Paleo life simple, always keep a dozen hard-boiled eggs in your refrigerator at any given time. They make quick snacks and great salad toppers, and they can be refrigerated up to 1 week.

1. In a prewarmed medium skillet over medium heat, cook bacon until done, about 4 minutes on each side. Set bacon aside, but leave drippings in pan. Add shrimp to skillet along with water, oil, lemon juice, salt, and pepper. Cook shrimp until pink, about 4 minutes.

2. In 2 large salad bowls, evenly divide greens, tomatoes, and eggs. Crumble bacon and split between bowls. Divide shrimp between bowls. Serve immediately with salad dressing of choice or refrigerate for use the next day. Keep in refrigerator up to 1 day.

Per Serving Calories: 392 | Fat: 27g | Protein: 22g | Sodium: 1,043mg | Fiber: 3g | Carbohydrates: 13g | Sugar: 8g

Salmon Cabbage Salad

This salad is rich in omega-3 fatty acids, making it an anti-inflammatory powerhouse.

PREP TIME: 10 MINUTES
COOK TIME: 10–15 MINUTES

INGREDIENTS | SERVES 2

2 (6-ounce) salmon fillets, thawed or fresh

1 teaspoon fine sea salt

½ teaspoon ground black pepper

2 tablespoons ghee

2 tablespoons avocado oil

1 tablespoon coconut aminos

½ tablespoon lemon juice

2 teaspoons raw honey

½ medium head purple cabbage, shredded

½ medium head green cabbage, shredded

3 large carrots, peeled and shredded

1 small yellow onion, peeled and diced

2 tablespoons whole raw hemp seeds

1. Preheat oven to 375°F. Line a baking sheet with foil. Place salmon fillets on foiled sheet and brush with salt, pepper, and ghee. Bake 10–15 minutes or until center of salmon flakes easily with fork. Remove from heat.

2. In a small mixing bowl, whisk together oil, coconut aminos, lemon juice, and honey. Set aside.

3. In a large mixing bowl, toss together cabbage, carrots, and onion. Drizzle with avocado oil mixture and stir to evenly coat mixture. Separate into 2 serving bowls, place 1 salmon fillet on each, and top with hemp seeds.

Per Serving   Calories: 839 | Fat: 39g | Protein: 49g | Sodium: 1,580mg | Fiber: 23g | Carbohydrates: 73g | Sugar: 42g

Salmon Quality Matters

When it comes to selecting the most nutritious fish, always choose wild-caught varieties. These will come in different forms, but the most common is wild-caught Alaskan pink salmon.

Sautéed Pepper Salad

This simple dish can be served warm or cold and will keep in the refrigerator up to 3 days.
Cook it up ahead of time for a party or picnic.

PREP TIME: 10 MINUTES
COOK TIME: 10 MINUTES

INGREDIENTS | SERVES 4

1 large red bell pepper, seeded and thinly sliced

1 large orange bell pepper, seeded and thinly sliced

1 large green bell pepper, seeded and thinly sliced

1 large yellow bell pepper, seeded and thinly sliced

1 small yellow onion, peeled and thinly sliced

2 cups grape tomatoes, halved

½ teaspoon fine sea salt

2 tablespoons lemon juice

1 tablespoon apple cider vinegar

1 tablespoon avocado oil

In a large skillet over medium-high heat, add all ingredients and sauté until peppers are softened and starting to blacken at edges, about 10 minutes. Remove from heat and serve warm or refrigerate in an airtight container and serve cold.

Per Serving   Calories: 91 | Fat: 3.5g | Protein: 2g | Sodium: 290mg | Fiber: 4g | Carbohydrates: 12g | Sugar: 7g

Super Green Salad

*This cold salad tastes best when made a day in advance
so that the vegetables can soak up the dressing.*

PREP TIME: 1 DAY
COOK TIME: N/A

INGREDIENTS | SERVES 4

2 large zucchini, spiralized

1 cup baby spinach

1 cup finely chopped chard

1 cup finely chopped beet greens

12 small radishes, trimmed and quartered

2 tablespoons avocado oil

½ teaspoon fine sea salt

⅛ teaspoon ground black pepper

½ teaspoon garlic powder

3 green onions, finely chopped

Stir together all ingredients in a medium glass mixing bowl. Cover and refrigerate 1 day. Serve chilled.

Per Serving Calories: 89 | Fat: 7g | Protein: 2g | Sodium: 335mg | Fiber: 2g | Carbohydrates: 5g | Sugar: 3g

Radishes

Radishes are yet another member of the popular category of vegetables known as cruciferous. While many will say that these should be avoided if thyroid disease is present, the benefits of eating this family of vegetables far outweigh any possible negative effects.

Kitchen Sink Slaw

*You can make this slaw with just about any vegetables you have on hand,
and even though it's ideally made with a food processor or a spiralizer,
you can also prep it using a grater, peeler, or even just by chopping with a sharp knife.*

PREP TIME: 1 HOUR 30 MINUTES
COOK TIME: N/A

INGREDIENTS | SERVES 8

1 large red onion, peeled and spiralized or pulsed

4 large carrots, peeled and spiralized or pulsed

1 medium head purple cabbage, grated or pulsed

2 medium Golden Delicious apples, peeled and spiralized or pulsed

3 tablespoons lemon juice

¼ cup Homemade Mayonnaise (see recipe in Chapter 16)

½ teaspoon coarse Himalayan salt

⅛ teaspoon ground black pepper

¼ teaspoon garlic powder

Combine all ingredients in a large glass dish, stirring well to make sure all vegetables are evenly coated. Cover and refrigerate about 1 hour. Serve chilled. Store in refrigerator for up to 3 days.

Per Serving Calories: 123 | Fat: 7g | Protein: 2g | Sodium: 138mg | Fiber: 4g | Carbohydrates: 15g | Sugar: 9g

Cucumber Salad

*This simple dish has only 4 ingredients and is an
easy side that can be thrown together in just a few minutes.*

PREP TIME: 5 MINUTES
COOK TIME: N/A

INGREDIENTS | SERVES 4

3 large cucumbers, finely chopped

1 tablespoon avocado oil

1 tablespoon lemon juice

½ teaspoon fine sea salt

Stir together all ingredients in a medium bowl. Serve immediately or keep in refrigerator up to 2 days.

Per Serving Calories: 59 | Fat: 3g | Protein: 1g | Sodium: 284mg | Fiber: 1.5g | Carbohydrates: 5g | Sugar: 3g

Cucumbers as Digestive Aids

When this salad is eaten before a high-protein meal, the cucumbers will actually help your body digest protein better, thanks to an enzyme known as erepsin. Cucumbers also help prevent water retention, and thus are a popular weight-loss food.

Super Green Superfood Salad

The name of the game with this salad is all green, all day long.
Even the light dressing is green thanks to the avocado oil.

PREP TIME: 20 MINUTES
COOK TIME: N/A

INGREDIENTS | SERVES 2

2 cups baby spinach

1 cup coarsely chopped arugula

1 cup coarsely torn romaine lettuce

1 cup coarsely chopped chard

1 cup finely chopped green cabbage

4 green onions, chopped

2 medium Granny Smith apples, diced

½ cup green grapes, halved

¼ cup pumpkin seeds

1 medium cucumber, thinly sliced

2 cups diced broccoli florets

3 tablespoons avocado oil

1 tablespoon lemon juice

1 tablespoon lime juice

½ teaspoon fine sea salt

1 medium avocado, pitted, peeled, and sliced

In a large salad bowl, toss together all ingredients except avocado. Once thoroughly mixed, top with avocado slices and serve immediately.

Per Serving Calories: 586 | Fat: 36g | Protein: 12g | Sodium: 676mg | Fiber: 17g | Carbohydrates: 53g | Sugar: 28g

Chicken Bacon Salad

Serve this as a side dish or as a meal wrapped in lettuce or topped on a bed of fresh, leafy greens.

PREP TIME: 15 MINUTES
COOK TIME: 35 MINUTES

INGREDIENTS | SERVES 4

3 (4-ounce) boneless, skinless chicken breasts

1 teaspoon sea salt, divided

1 cup Chicken Stock (see recipe in Chapter 6)

6 green onions, sliced

½ cup bacon crumbles

¼ cup Homemade Mayonnaise (see recipe in Chapter 16)

1 tablespoon lemon juice

¼ teaspoon ground black pepper

1 teaspoon garlic powder

1. Preheat oven to 375°F. Place chicken breasts, ½ teaspoon sea salt, and stock in a medium glass baking dish. Bake uncovered 35 minutes or until center of chicken reaches an internal temperature of 165°F.

2. In a medium mixing bowl, combine remaining ingredients. Shred chicken with a fork and stir into mixture. Serve immediately or chill before serving. Keep in refrigerator up to 3 days.

Per Serving   Calories: 306 | Fat: 19.5g | Protein: 26g | Sodium: 1,188mg | Fiber: 0.5g | Carbohydrates: 2g | Sugar: 0.5g

Apple Salad with Bacon and Almonds

This sweet dish is best served as an appetizer or on a bed of mixed leafy greens.

PREP TIME: 10 MINUTES
COOK TIME: 8 MINUTES

INGREDIENTS | SERVES 4

10 slices bacon, cut into 1" pieces

1 large Granny Smith apple, cored and diced

1 large Honeycrisp apple, cored and diced

1 large Golden Delicious apple, cored and diced

⅔ cup almond slivers

½ teaspoon coarse Himalayan salt

1 tablespoon lemon juice

1. In a large skillet over medium heat, cook bacon until crispy, turning often, about 8 minutes. Remove bacon and set aside. Transfer bacon drippings to a medium mixing bowl.

2. Add remaining ingredients to bacon drippings and stir well. Top with bacon pieces and serve immediately, or keep in refrigerator up to 1 day.

Per Serving   Calories: 293 | Fat: 19g | Protein: 14g | Sodium: 680mg | Fiber: 3g | Carbohydrates: 18.5g | Sugar: 12g

Ginger Apple Chicken Salad

Serve this savory chicken salad dish with Paleo bread,
lettuce wraps, or a side of Jicama "Rice" (see recipe in Chapter 13).

PREP TIME: 20 MINUTES
COOK TIME: 30 MINUTES

INGREDIENTS | SERVES 4

3 (6-ounce) boneless, skinless chicken breasts

1 cup Chicken Stock (see recipe in Chapter 6)

1 teaspoon coarse Himalayan salt, divided

¼ teaspoon ground black pepper

¼ teaspoon paprika

⅛ teaspoon red pepper flakes

½ large pineapple, peeled, cored, and diced

½ medium head green cabbage, shredded

¼ cup Homemade Mayonnaise (see recipe in Chapter 16)

1 tablespoon lemon juice

½ teaspoon ground ginger

1 large Granny Smith apple, cored and diced

3 green onions, sliced

1. Preheat oven to 375°F. Place chicken in a medium glass baking dish and add stock and ½ teaspoon salt. Bake uncovered until internal temperature of chicken reaches 165°F, about 30 minutes.

2. In a large mixing bowl stir together remaining ingredients. Cut chicken into chunks and add to bowl. Serve immediately or refrigerate up to 3 days.

Per Serving Calories: 356 | Fat: 16g | Protein: 30g | Sodium: 523mg | Fiber: 4g | Carbohydrates: 21g | Sugar: 12g

Why Himalayan Salt?

There are several different varieties of sea salt, but Himalayan salt is actually health supportive for endocrine function, including thyroid and adrenal glands. The pink hue of the salt comes from mineral content—specifically, it is rich in iron.

Tangy Asian Pork Salad

*This quick one-dish meal is perfect for lunch on the go,
or served as an appetizer before a stir-fry dinner.*

PREP TIME: 20 MINUTES
COOK TIME: 5–7 MINUTES

INGREDIENTS | SERVES 4

3 tablespoons coconut aminos

½ tablespoon Worcestershire sauce

1 tablespoon avocado oil

1 large lemon, juiced

1 small lime, juiced

3 clementines, peeled and separated

½ tablespoon minced garlic

1 tablespoon coconut oil

4 (4-ounce) boneless pork chops, cubed

1 large yellow bell pepper, seeded and thinly sliced

1 medium head green cabbage, shredded

6 green onions, sliced

¼ cup slivered almonds

1. In a large skillet or wok, toss together all ingredients except cabbage, onions, and almonds. Sauté, stirring frequently, over medium-high heat until pork is no longer pink, about 5–7 minutes. Remove from heat.

2. Divide cabbage equally among 4 serving bowls and tops with onions. Spoon out equal portions of pork mixture and top with slivered almonds. Serve warm.

Per Serving   Calories: 332 | Fat: 13g | Protein: 29g | Sodium: 627mg | Fiber: 6.5g | Carbohydrates: 25.5g | Sugar: 6g

Roasted Radish Salad

If you're not usually a fan of radishes because of their sulfuric taste, this method of cooking will not only make them sweeter, but is also ideal for an alternative form of salad topping.

PREP TIME: 15 MINUTES
COOK TIME: 35 MINUTES

INGREDIENTS | SERVES 4

2 pounds radishes, trimmed and halved

3 tablespoons avocado oil

2 tablespoons red wine vinegar

¼ teaspoon ground black pepper

1 teaspoon coarse Himalayan salt

1 tablespoon minced garlic

1 medium red onion, peeled and thinly sliced

¼ cup apple cider vinegar

1 large red apple, cored and thinly sliced

Preheat oven to 425°F. In a medium mixing bowl, toss together all ingredients. Spread evenly across a baking sheet. Bake 35 minutes or until radishes are tender and easily pierced with a fork. Serve warm or keep chilled in refrigerator up to 3 days.

Per Serving Calories: 143 | Fat: 8.5g | Protein: 1.5g | Sodium: 437mg | Fiber: 3.5g | Carbohydrates: 15g | Sugar: 9g

Avocado Salad

This simple no-cook dish works great on its own or paired with leafy greens or cabbage.

PREP TIME: 5 MINUTES
COOK TIME: N/A

INGREDIENTS | SERVES 4

3 ripe avocados, pitted, peeled, and thinly sliced

1½ cups grape tomatoes, halved

1 teaspoon coarse Himalayan salt

3 tablespoons ghee

2 green onions, sliced

1. In 4 serving bowls, evenly place avocado slices, then top with tomatoes.

2. In a small mixing bowl, stir together salt and ghee. Drizzle mixture over avocado and tomatoes and top with green onions. Serve immediately.

Per Serving Calories: 283 | Fat: 25g | Protein: 3g | Sodium: 392mg | Fiber: 8g | Carbohydrates: 11g | Sugar: 1g

Beet Green Salad

When roasting beets for a different recipe, save the greens and turn them into a delicious salad!

PREP TIME: 10 MINUTES
COOK TIME: N/A

INGREDIENTS | SERVES 4

4 cups chopped beet greens

2 cups baby spinach

1 cup chopped dandelion greens

1 cup chopped Swiss chard

4 large hard-boiled eggs, peeled and sliced

1 large carrot, peeled and shredded

1 cup thinly sliced portobello mushrooms

½ cup Avocado Vinaigrette (see recipe in Chapter 16)

Toss together all ingredients except Avocado Vinaigrette in a large mixing bowl. Drizzle with Avocado Vinaigrette and serve immediately or chill up to 4 hours.

Per Serving Calories: 424 | Fat: 36g | Protein: 10g | Sodium: 344mg | Fiber: 5g | Carbohydrates: 15g | Sugar: 6.5g

Asian Broccoli Slaw

This dish works perfectly served cold, but for a change of pace, throw it in a wok or skillet and sauté until warm.

PREP TIME: 15 MINUTES
COOK TIME: N/A

INGREDIENTS | SERVES 4

2 large heads broccoli, florets separated and finely chopped

1 small red onion, peeled and finely chopped

1 large carrot, peeled and shredded

½ medium head green cabbage, shredded

¼ cup coconut aminos

½ tablespoon fish sauce

1 tablespoon lemon juice

½ teaspoon coarse Himalayan salt

Stir together all ingredients and serve immediately or refrigerate up to 2 days.

Per Serving Calories: 116 | Fat: 0.3g | Protein: 7g | Sodium: 704mg | Fiber: 8g | Carbohydrates: 24g | Sugar: 5g

Sweet Potato Salad

Cook this salad ahead of time and reheat to serve, or serve chilled with any meat. Also pairs well with eggs or breakfast meats.

PREP TIME: 10 MINUTES
COOK TIME: 40 MINUTES

INGREDIENTS | SERVES 4

3 large sweet potatoes, peeled and cubed

2 tablespoons coconut oil

1 teaspoon fine sea salt

¼ teaspoon ground black pepper

½ cup slivered walnuts

⅓ cup lemon juice

2 tablespoons raw honey

2 tablespoons minced onion

4 cups baby spinach

1. Preheat oven to 400°F. In a large mixing bowl, toss together all ingredients except spinach. Spread evenly on a baking sheet and bake 35 minutes.

2. Remove from oven, spread spinach across mixture, and return to oven 5 minutes or until spinach starts to wilt. Serve warm or chilled.

Per Serving Calories: 303 | Fat: 16g | Protein: 5.5g | Sodium: 622mg | Fiber: 5g | Carbohydrates: 36g | Sugar: 17g

Beet, Apple, and Bacon Slaw

Use this dish as an appetizer or a side, paired with a meal that is red-meat focused.

PREP TIME: 45 MINUTES
COOK TIME: N/A

INGREDIENTS | SERVES 4

3 tablespoons avocado oil

2 tablespoons apple cider vinegar

1 tablespoon lemon juice

1 teaspoon garlic powder

¼ teaspoon fine sea salt

2 clementines, peeled and separated

6 slices bacon, cooked and crumbled

1 large beet, peeled and shredded, greens finely chopped

1 large Granny Smith apple, cored and shredded

1 small jicama, peeled and shredded

1 large carrot, peeled and shredded

In a large mixing bowl, toss together all ingredients. Chill 30 minutes before serving. Keep in refrigerator up to 3 days.

Per Serving Calories: 265 | Fat: 16g | Protein: 7g | Sodium: 459mg | Fiber: 6.5g | Carbohydrates: 23g | Sugar: 12g

Salmon Salad with Garlic

Get your omega-3s in easily with this delicious, creamy salad that pairs well with Paleo bread or a huge pile of leafy greens. Serve it on a side salad with baked salmon for a "salmon two ways" spread that will be effortlessly gourmet.

PREP TIME: 5 MINUTES
COOK TIME: N/A

INGREDIENTS | SERVES 2

2 (6-ounce) cans wild-caught salmon, drained

¼ cup Homemade Mayonnaise (see recipe in Chapter 16)

½ teaspoon fine sea salt

¼ teaspoon ground black pepper

¼ teaspoon onion powder

¼ teaspoon garlic powder

2 green onions, sliced

2 teaspoons lemon juice

In a medium bowl, flake apart salmon with a fork. Stir in remaining ingredients until well combined. Serve immediately or refrigerate up to 1 day before using.

Per Serving Calories: 473 | Fat: 34g | Protein: 34.5g | Sodium: 1,176mg | Fiber: 0.3g | Carbohydrates: 2g | Sugar: 0.4g

Pineapple Salad

This sweet and hot dish pairs nicely with whitefish or poultry. Prep it a day ahead for convenience.

PREP TIME: 1 HOUR
COOK TIME: N/A

INGREDIENTS | SERVES 4

1 large pineapple, peeled, cored, and diced

1 small jicama, peeled and grated

1 small red onion, peeled and grated

1 small red apple, cored and grated

3 tablespoons avocado oil

1 tablespoon lemon juice

¼ teaspoon fine sea salt

⅛ teaspoon cayenne pepper

In a medium mixing bowl, stir together all ingredients. Refrigerate 30–40 minutes to chill before serving, or make ahead. Store in refrigerator for up to 2 days.

Per Serving Calories: 207 | Fat: 10g | Protein: 1.5g | Sodium: 144mg | Fiber: 6g | Carbohydrates: 29g | Sugar: 17g

Floret Salad

Broccoli is one of the most nutrient-dense green vegetables.
Try this floret salad to maximize on taste while boosting your health simultaneously.

PREP TIME: 5 MINUTES
COOK TIME: N/A

INGREDIENTS | SERVES 2

⅔ cup fresh cauliflower florets
⅔ cup fresh broccoli florets
2 tablespoons chopped red onion
8 ounces bacon, cooked and chopped
5 teaspoons raw honey
¼ cup walnut oil
2 tablespoons whole cashews

1. In a medium bowl, combine cauliflower, broccoli, onion, and bacon.

2. In a small bowl, whisk together honey and walnut oil.

3. Combine honey mixture with florets and toss.

4. Top with cashews just before serving.

Per Serving Calories: 749 | Fat: 62g | Protein: 29g | Sodium: 884mg | Fiber: 2g | Carbohydrates: 22g | Sugar: 16g

Broccoli: Superfood

Broccoli is one of the healthiest vegetables you can eat. Ounce for ounce, broccoli has more vitamin C than an orange and as much calcium as a glass of milk. Broccoli is packed with fiber to promote digestive health and it is quite rich in vitamin A.

Beet and Cauliflower Salad

Beets are a great source of antioxidants that help reduce the risk of cancer.
They are also a great source of folate, magnesium, and potassium.
Just remember to wear gloves when you work with beets, or your hands will be stained red for days.

PREP TIME: 30 MINUTES
COOK TIME: 65–75 MINUTES

INGREDIENTS | SERVES 4

4 large beets
½ cup water
¼ cup extra-virgin olive oil
1 medium shallot, peeled and minced
2 tablespoons apple cider vinegar
2 tablespoons full-fat coconut milk
1 tablespoon Grade B maple syrup
½ teaspoon sea salt
⅛ teaspoon ground black pepper
6 cups mixed salad greens
1 large head cauliflower, cut into florets
½ cup toasted pumpkin or sunflower seeds
½ cup sliced fresh basil leaves

1. Preheat oven to 375°F. Place beets in a medium baking dish. Add water, cover tightly with foil, and bake about 65–75 minutes or until beets are pierced easily with a knife. Remove from baking dish and let cool on wire rack for 20 minutes.

2. When beets are cool, peel and cut into ½" cubes. Set aside.

3. In a medium salad bowl, combine oil, shallot, vinegar, coconut milk, maple syrup, salt, and pepper and mix well.

4. Add greens and beets and toss to coat.

5. Top with cauliflower florets, seeds, and basil and serve immediately.

Per Serving   Calories: 283 | Fat: 21g | Protein: 8g | Sodium: 417mg | Fiber: 5g | Carbohydrates: 19g | Sugar: 9g

Celeriac Slaw

Celeriac is a vegetable in the celery family.
You can pair this slaw with most meat, fish, or poultry for a tasty counterpoint.

PREP TIME: 5 MINUTES
COOK TIME: N/A

INGREDIENTS | SERVES 6

1 bulb celeriac, peeled and coarsely grated

1 tablespoon Homemade Mayonnaise (see recipe in Chapter 16)

1 tablespoon white wine vinegar

¼ teaspoon dried thyme

½ teaspoon sea salt

½ teaspoon ground black pepper

1 teaspoon dry mustard

Place celeriac in a medium bowl. In a small bowl, mix together mayonnaise, vinegar, thyme, salt, pepper, and mustard. Pour over celeriac and mix to combine. Serve immediately or chill for up to 1 day before serving.

Per Serving   Calories: 46 | Fat: 2.5g | Protein: 1g | Sodium: 251mg | Fiber: 1g | Carbohydrates: 5.5g | Sugar: 1g

Curried Chicken Salad

The recipe makes 2 servings, but you can easily double or triple it.
You can also change the spices around for more variety.

PREP TIME: 25 MINUTES
COOK TIME: 10 MINUTES

INGREDIENTS | SERVES 2

2 tablespoons almond oil

8 ounces chicken breast, cubed

1 medium stalk celery, sliced

1 small onion, peeled and diced

½ English cucumber, diced

½ cup chopped almonds

2 medium apples, peeled, cored, and chopped

½ teaspoon curry powder

4 cups baby romaine lettuce

1. In frying pan, heat oil over medium-high heat and cook chicken, celery, and onion about 10 minutes or until chicken is cooked through. Set aside to cool.

2. In mixing bowl, combine cucumber, almonds, apples, and curry powder with cooled chicken mixture.

3. Serve over a bed of baby romaine lettuce.

Per Serving   Calories: 460 | Fat: 23g | Protein: 31.5g | Sodium: 25mg | Fiber: 9g | Carbohydrates: 34g | Sugar: 21g

Arugula and Fennel Salad with Pomegranate

Pomegranates pack a high dose of health-promoting antioxidants.
They are in peak season October through January and may not be easy to find at other times of the year.
Cranberries can be substituted in this recipe if pomegranates are not available.

PREP TIME: 15 MINUTES
COOK TIME: N/A

INGREDIENTS | SERVES 4

4 cups arugula

2 large navel oranges, peeled and cut into 10–12 pieces each

Seeds of 1 large pomegranate

1 cup thinly sliced fennel

¼ cup extra-virgin olive oil

¼ teaspoon sea salt

¼ teaspoon ground black pepper

1. Place arugula, oranges, pomegranate seeds, and fennel in a large bowl.

2. Toss salad with oil, salt, and pepper to coat evenly. Serve immediately or refrigerate for up to 1 day.

Per Serving   Calories: 195 | Fat: 13g | Protein: 2g | Sodium: 163mg | Fiber: 4g | Carbohydrates: 18g | Sugar: 13g

Filet Mignon and Red Onion Salad

There are few things that taste better cold than filet mignon!

PREP TIME: 25 MINUTES
COOK TIME: 15 MINUTES

INGREDIENTS | SERVES 4

1¼ pounds well-trimmed whole filet mignon

¼ teaspoon sea salt

¼ teaspoon ground black pepper

½ cup French Dressing (see recipe in Chapter 16)

1 large red onion, peeled and thinly sliced

2 tablespoons capers, rinsed and drained

16 black olives, pitted and sliced

8 cups chopped romaine lettuce

1. Preheat oven to 400°F. Place filet mignon in a baking pan. Sprinkle with salt and pepper. Roast 15 minutes. Let meat rest 10 minutes.

2. Slice filet mignon and place in a medium bowl with dressing, onion, capers, and olives. Toss gently to coat.

3. Spread lettuce on a serving platter. Arrange filet mignon mixture over top. Serve at room temperature or chilled.

Per Serving   Calories: 413 | Fat: 27g | Protein: 32g | Sodium: 370mg | Fiber: 3g | Carbohydrates: 8g | Sugar: 3g

CHAPTER 13

Side Dishes

Roasted Tomatoes, Peppers, and Green Beans

This simple side dish can be thrown together in a pinch and can easily be modified to include whatever vegetables you have on hand.

PREP TIME: 10 MINUTES
COOK TIME: 20–25 MINUTES

INGREDIENTS | SERVES 4

8 medium Roma tomatoes, halved lengthwise

2 teaspoons fine sea salt, divided

1 large green bell pepper, seeded and sliced

1 large red bell pepper, seeded and sliced

1 large yellow bell pepper, seeded and sliced

2 cups green beans, trimmed

¼ teaspoon ground black pepper

1 tablespoon avocado oil

1 tablespoon minced garlic

1 large lemon, juiced

2 large lemons, cut into wedges

Keep It Cool

Try serving this dish chilled as a Paleo alternative to pasta salad. It'll make the perfect addition to any picnic, carry-in dinner, or family-style meal.

1. Preheat oven to 450°F. Line a baking sheet with foil. Evenly space tomatoes on baking sheet skin side down. Sprinkle with 1 teaspoon salt. Bake 5 minutes.

2. Meanwhile, in a medium mixing bowl toss together peppers, green beans, remaining salt, pepper, oil, garlic, and lemon juice until vegetables are evenly coated. Spread on baking sheet around tomatoes. Cover entire baking sheet with foil and return to oven.

3. Bake 15–20 minutes or until green beans are softened. Garnish with lemon wedges and serve warm.

Per Serving Calories: 154 | Fat: 5.5g | Protein: 4g | Sodium: 995mg | Fiber: 5g | Carbohydrates: 24g | Sugar: 14g

Garlic-Sautéed Green Beans and Portobellos

*This garlicky side dish pairs perfectly with any red meat and
even works alongside eggs for a savory breakfast combo.*

PREP TIME: 5 MINUTES
COOK TIME: 10 MINUTES

INGREDIENTS | SERVES 4

2 pounds green beans, trimmed

2 tablespoons avocado oil

2 tablespoons ghee

4 cloves garlic, peeled and chopped

1 pound portobello mushrooms, sliced

½ teaspoon fine sea salt

¼ teaspoon ground black pepper

¼ teaspoon onion powder

½ teaspoon garlic powder

In a large frying pan over medium-high heat, add all ingredients and sauté until green beans are softened, about 10 minutes. Stir frequently. Serve warm.

Per Serving   Calories: 210 | Fat: 13g | Protein: 6g | Sodium: 302mg | Fiber: 9g | Carbohydrates: 20g | Sugar: 3g

Roasted Kohlrabi

A less popular root vegetable, kohlrabi is similar in flavor to turnips or parsnips.

PREP TIME: 10 MINUTES
COOK TIME: 20 MINUTES

INGREDIENTS | SERVES 4

8 kohlrabi bulbs, peeled and sliced

2 tablespoons avocado oil

¼ teaspoon fine sea salt

¼ teaspoon onion powder

¼ teaspoon garlic powder

1. Preheat oven to 350°F. Line a baking sheet with foil.

2. Spread kohlrabi slices evenly across the sheet so they don't overlap. (Depending on the diameter of the bulbs, this may take 2 trays.) Evenly brush slices with avocado oil and sprinkle with seasonings. Bake 20 minutes or until edges crisp and kohlrabi starts to brown. Serve warm.

Per Serving   Calories: 127 | Fat: 7g | Protein: 4g | Sodium: 187mg | Fiber: 9g | Carbohydrates: 15g | Sugar: 6g

Skillet-Cooked Vegetables with Lemon

This tasty blend of several vegetables and greens makes for the perfect side dish to pair with any meat or main dish. Add some bacon to the skillet for a tasty breakfast alternative.

PREP TIME: 20 MINUTES
COOK TIME: 30 MINUTES

INGREDIENTS | SERVES 4

6 ounces baby beets, halved and greens chopped

1 small sweet onion, peeled and chopped

6 ounces fingerling potatoes, halved

1 small parsnip, peeled and chopped

3 tablespoons avocado oil

1 cup sugar snap peas, trimmed

½ teaspoon fine sea salt

⅛ teaspoon ground black pepper

1 teaspoon onion powder

1 teaspoon garlic powder

2 large lemons, juiced

1 cup baby spinach

4 heads baby bok choy, trimmed and chopped

1. In a large skillet over medium heat, cook beets, onion, potatoes, and parsnip in avocado oil 12 minutes, covered and stirring every 2–3 minutes. Remove lid and cook an additional 10 minutes or until beets are soft enough to spear with a fork.

2. Add peas, seasonings, and lemon juice to skillet and cook 3–4 minutes or until peas turn brighter green and begin to soften. Add spinach, bok choy, and beet greens and cook another 2–3 minutes or until spinach begins to wilt, stirring frequently. Remove from heat and serve.

Per Serving   Calories: 271 | Fat: 11g | Protein: 12g | Sodium: 716mg | Fiber: 10.5g | Carbohydrates: 36g | Sugar: 13g

Greens and Garlic

This dark green skillet blend is the perfect way to get in your daily calcium, as well as folate and vitamin C.

PREP TIME: 10 MINUTES
COOK TIME: 20 MINUTES

INGREDIENTS | SERVES 4

4 cloves garlic, peeled and chopped

3 tablespoons avocado oil

1 large head broccoli, florets separated and stem finely chopped

2 cups coarsely torn kale

2 cups coarsely chopped chard

1 large fennel bulb, coarsely chopped

15 spears asparagus, ends trimmed, chopped

1 teaspoon fine sea salt

¼ teaspoon ground black pepper

¼ cup lemon juice

1. In a large skillet over medium-high heat, sauté garlic in oil 5–7 minutes or until aromatic. Add broccoli florets and stem and sauté an additional 5–7 minutes.

2. Add remaining ingredients to skillet and sauté 7 minutes or until leafy greens have wilted and asparagus has turned bright green, stirring frequently. Remove from heat and serve immediately.

Per Serving Calories: 187 | Fat: 9g | Protein: 7g | Sodium: 683mg | Fiber: 8g | Carbohydrates: 20g | Sugar: 7g

Candied Carrots

This super easy roast vegetable dish will be a favorite. The flavors are reminiscent of carrot cake, and thus this dish can double as both side and dessert. It is a great alternative to non-Paleo versions of sweet potatoes slathered with marshmallows and caramel sauce.

PREP TIME: 5 MINUTES
COOK TIME: 35–40 MINUTES

INGREDIENTS | SERVES 4

8 large carrots, peeled, halved, and cut into 3" sticks

2 tablespoons coconut oil

1 tablespoon coconut sugar

½ teaspoon ground cinnamon

⅛ teaspoon ground nutmeg

⅛ teaspoon ground ginger

⅛ teaspoon fine sea salt

1. Preheat oven to 375°F. Line a baking sheet with foil.

2. In a small mixing bowl, toss together all ingredients and spread evenly on baking sheet. Bake 35–40 minutes or until carrots are soft and easily speared with a fork. Serve warm.

Per Serving Calories: 130 | Fat: 7g | Protein: 1g | Sodium: 169mg | Fiber: 4g | Carbohydrates: 17g | Sugar: 10g

Slow-Cooked Radishes and Roots

Let your slow cooker do the work with this easily prepped side dish that pairs nicely with beef or chicken.

PREP TIME: 10 MINUTES
COOK TIME: 2–6 HOURS

INGREDIENTS | SERVES 4

2 pounds radishes, trimmed and halved

4 large carrots, peeled and sliced

1 small yellow onion, peeled and sliced

1 fennel bulb, trimmed and sliced

1 large beet, peeled and sliced

6 cloves garlic, peeled and quartered

3 cups Chicken Stock (see recipe in Chapter 6)

1 teaspoon fine sea salt

½ teaspoon ground black pepper

Place all ingredients in a 4- or 6-quart slow cooker. Ensure that at least half the vegetables are covered with stock. If necessary, add water to reach that level. Cover and cook on high 2–3 hours or on low 5–6 hours. Serve warm.

Per Serving Calories: 151 | Fat: 4g | Protein: 6g | Sodium: 1,097mg | Fiber: 9g | Carbohydrates: 24.5g | Sugar: 12g

Spicy Potatoes

This easy side dish is cooked in a slow cooker to produce the softest, melt-in-your-mouth potatoes you've ever tasted. Serve alongside chicken, beef, or fish.

PREP TIME: 5 MINUTES
COOK TIME: 3–7 HOURS

INGREDIENTS | SERVES 4

2 pounds small fingerling potatoes, halved

4 cups Chicken Stock (see recipe in Chapter 6)

1 teaspoon fine sea salt

½ teaspoon ground black pepper

2 teaspoons yellow mustard

2 teaspoons garlic powder

1 teaspoon onion powder

⅛ teaspoon cayenne pepper

2 medium stalks celery, diced

Add all ingredients to a 4- or 6-quart slow cooker. Cover and cook on high 3–4 hours or on low 6–7 hours. Serve warm. Can be kept in refrigerator up to 3 days.

Per Serving Calories: 265 | Fat: 4g | Protein: 9g | Sodium: 1,105mg | Fiber: 4g | Carbohydrates: 45g | Sugar: 1g

Buttery Steamed Asparagus

With just 4 ingredients, this simple yet satisfying side is perfectly paired with any main dish. Use leftovers with eggs for a quick breakfast dish!

PREP TIME: 5 MINUTES
COOK TIME: 12–15 MINUTES

INGREDIENTS | SERVES 4

32 spears asparagus, ends trimmed off
1 teaspoon coarse Himalayan salt
3 tablespoons ghee
1 tablespoon water

1. Preheat oven to 400°F. Line a baking sheet with foil.

2. Lay asparagus on baking sheet in a single row and sprinkle with salt. Spoon ghee and water on top of the asparagus. Cover with foil, leaving one end open for steam to escape. Bake 12–15 minutes or until asparagus is pierced easily with a fork. Serve warm.

Per Serving   Calories: 93 | Fat: 8g | Protein: 3g | Sodium: 382mg | Fiber: 3g | Carbohydrates: 5g | Sugar: 2g

Asparagus Health Benefits

Asparagus is a low-carb vegetable and is also an extremely rich source of vitamin K, folate, and copper—all essential for total body wellness and optimal thyroid function. It also supports blood sugar regulation, as well as proper digestion.

Lemon-Roasted Broccoli Raab

This delicious leafy green tastes much sweeter when roasted to the point of crispness—so good that you'll want to load up your plate with seconds.

PREP TIME: 5 MINUTES
COOK TIME: 8–10 MINUTES

INGREDIENTS | SERVES 4

1 large bunch broccoli raab, stems removed
¼ cup avocado oil
2 large lemons, juiced
½ teaspoon coarse Himalayan salt
¼ teaspoon ground black pepper
1 tablespoon minced garlic

Preheat oven to 400°F. Line a baking sheet with foil. Spread broccoli raab evenly across baking sheet. Drizzle with oil and lemon juice. Sprinkle with salt, pepper, and garlic. Bake 8–10 minutes or until starting to crisp. Serve warm.

Per Serving   Calories: 101 | Fat: 10g | Protein: 0.5g | Sodium: 193mg | Fiber: 0.4g | Carbohydrates: 2g | Sugar: 0.4g

Roasted Cauliflower

This simple side can fill the "potatoes" slot in any meat-and-potatoes meal.

PREP TIME: 10 MINUTES
COOK TIME: 30 MINUTES

INGREDIENTS | SERVES 4

2 large heads cauliflower, florets separated into 1" sections

¼ cup ghee

2 tablespoons avocado oil

½ teaspoon fine sea salt

¼ teaspoon ground black pepper

¼ cup Chicken Stock (see recipe in Chapter 6)

Preheat oven to 400°F. In a large mixing bowl, toss together all ingredients until well mixed. Spread evenly on a baking sheet in a single layer and bake until cauliflower starts to brown and is soft when pierced with a fork, about 30 minutes.

Per Serving Calories: 261 | Fat: 22g | Protein: 5g | Sodium: 379mg | Fiber: 5g | Carbohydrates: 12g | Sugar: 4.5g

Spicy Lime Vegetables

Pair this dish with chicken or fish to add some extra pizzazz and color to your plate.

PREP TIME: 15 MINUTES
COOK TIME: 35 MINUTES

INGREDIENTS | SERVES 4

1 large turnip, peeled and cubed

1 large parsnip, peeled and cubed

1 large sweet potato, peeled and cubed

1 large red beet, peeled and cubed, greens reserved

1 small yellow onion, peeled and sliced

3 tablespoons avocado oil

½ teaspoon fine sea salt

¼ teaspoon ground black pepper

1 teaspoon ground chili pepper

⅛ teaspoon cayenne pepper

1 large lime, zested and juiced

1. Preheat oven to 450°F. Line a baking sheet with foil.

2. In a large mixing bowl, toss together all ingredients except beet greens. Spread evenly on baking sheet and cook 30 minutes. Remove from oven, add beet greens, and cook 5 more minutes. Serve warm.

Per Serving Calories: 174 | Fat: 10g | Protein: 2g | Sodium: 349mg | Fiber: 5g | Carbohydrates: 19g | Sugar: 7g

Honey-Roasted Parsnips

This dish can be made with any starchy root vegetable, including sweet potatoes, white potatoes, or even beets. Make things colorful by using a combination of them all.

PREP TIME: 10 MINUTES
COOK TIME: 35–40 MINUTES

INGREDIENTS | SERVES 4

4 large parsnips, peeled and cubed
¼ cup raw honey
2 tablespoons ghee
¼ teaspoon fine sea salt
⅛ teaspoon ground black pepper
½ teaspoon garlic powder

1. Preheat oven to 375°F. Line a baking sheet with foil.

2. In a large mixing bowl, toss together all ingredients, mixing thoroughly. Spread evenly across baking sheet. Cook 35–40 minutes or until vegetables are soft and pierced easily with a fork. Serve warm.

Per Serving Calories: 233 | Fat: 8g | Protein: 2g | Sodium: 153mg | Fiber: 7g | Carbohydrates: 41g | Sugar: 23g

Wilted Spinach

This simple 4-ingredient meal can be cooked using any dark leafy green for slightly different flavors. Or try a combination of several dark greens.

PREP TIME: 5 MINUTES
COOK TIME: 5 MINUTES

INGREDIENTS | SERVES 4

1 tablespoon lemon juice
2 tablespoons water
1 teaspoon fine sea salt
16 ounces baby spinach

In a large skillet over medium heat, warm lemon juice and water 1–2 minutes or until hot. Add salt and spinach, cover, and cook 2 minutes. Remove lid, stir, and cook an additional 1–2 minutes or until spinach is fully wilted. Serve warm.

Per Serving Calories: 31 | Fat: 0.3g | Protein: 3g | Sodium: 649mg | Fiber: 2.5g | Carbohydrates: 4g | Sugar: 1g

Roasted Zucchini Sticks

Missing chips or fries? These salty, crispy sticks are the perfect complement to any burger meal, and they make a tasty afternoon snack!

PREP TIME: 10 MINUTES
COOK TIME: 20 MINUTES

INGREDIENTS | SERVES 4

6 large zucchini, halved
½ cup avocado oil
2 teaspoons coarse Himalayan salt

1. Preheat oven to 475°F. Line a baking sheet with foil.

2. Take each zucchini half and slice into quarters, so that pieces resemble pickle spears. Lay out in a single layer on baking sheet. Brush each piece with avocado oil and sprinkle evenly with salt.

3. Bake 20 minutes or until strips are golden brown and edges are starting to crisp. Serve warm or cold.

Per Serving   Calories: 250 | Fat: 19g | Protein: 6g | Sodium: 741mg | Fiber: 5g | Carbohydrates: 15g | Sugar: 12g

Roasted Blackened Green Beans

This simple dish can be jazzed up by adding other flavors, including coconut aminos, cayenne pepper, or chili powder.

PREP TIME: 5 MINUTES
COOK TIME: 20 MINUTES

INGREDIENTS | SERVES 4

2 cups green beans, trimmed
3 tablespoons avocado oil
1 teaspoon coarse Himalayan salt
¼ teaspoon ground black pepper
3 tablespoons minced garlic
1 tablespoon lemon juice

1. Preheat oven to 425°F. Line a baking sheet with foil.

2. In a mixing bowl, combine all ingredients and stir to coat beans. Spread evenly on baking sheet and bake 20 minutes or until beans are soft and starting to blacken. Serve warm.

Per Serving   Calories: 118 | Fat: 10g | Protein: 1g | Sodium: 384mg | Fiber: 2g | Carbohydrates: 6g | Sugar: 0.2g

Sautéed Collard Greens

This quick and salty dish is tasty, simple, and the perfect complement to pork chops or any red meat.

PREP TIME: 5 MINUTES
COOK TIME: 8–10 MINUTES

INGREDIENTS | SERVES 4

4 cups collard greens, stems trimmed

2 tablespoons ghee

1 teaspoon fine sea salt

1 tablespoon minced garlic

In a large skillet over medium-high heat, toss together all ingredients and sauté 8–10 minutes or until collards are wilted and blackened, stirring frequently. Serve warm.

Per Serving   Calories: 87 | Fat: 8g | Protein: 1g | Sodium: 566mg | Fiber: 1.5g | Carbohydrates: 3g | Sugar: 0.2g

Chopped Zucchini and Peppers

This simple dish is cooked slightly, but still retains a salad-like crunch.

PREP TIME: 10 MINUTES
COOK TIME: 5 MINUTES

INGREDIENTS | SERVES 4

2 large zucchini, diced

1 large red bell pepper, seeded and diced

1 large yellow bell pepper, seeded and diced

1 small white onion, peeled and diced

2 tablespoons avocado oil

1 teaspoon garlic powder

½ teaspoon fine sea salt

In a large skillet over medium heat, stir together all ingredients and sauté about 5 minutes or until vegetables just start to soften. Serve warm or chilled.

Per Serving   Calories: 119 | Fat: 7g | Protein: 3g | Sodium: 295mg | Fiber: 3g | Carbohydrates: 11g | Sugar: 6g

Sautéed Turnip Greens

Reserve the greens from a different recipe using turnips so that no part gets wasted.

PREP TIME: 5 MINUTES
COOK TIME: 3 MINUTES

INGREDIENTS | SERVES 4

2 pounds turnip greens, roughly chopped

2 medium cloves garlic, peeled and smashed

1 tablespoon avocado oil

½ teaspoon fine sea salt

In a medium skillet over medium heat, toss together all ingredients and stir continuously 3 minutes. Remove from heat and serve immediately.

Per Serving Calories: 107 | Fat: 4g | Protein: 3.5g | Sodium: 370mg | Fiber: 7g | Carbohydrates: 17g | Sugar: 2g

Turnip Greens

Turnip greens have a slightly bitter taste that is due to their incredibly high mineral content, especially calcium and copper—both essential nutrients for proper thyroid function.

Okra Stuffed with Green Peppercorns

This is a delightful Indian dish. You can make it in advance and warm it up before serving. It's a great side dish for curry, and okra is a nice vegetable alternative if you get sick of the usual broccoli, asparagus, and zucchini.

PREP TIME: 5 MINUTES
COOK TIME: 10 MINUTES

INGREDIENTS | SERVES 2

½ cup Basic Vegetable Stock (see recipe in Chapter 6)

6 medium okra, stemmed

1 tablespoon brine-packed green peppercorns, rinsed and drained

1 teaspoon grassfed butter or ghee

1 teaspoon ground cumin

½ teaspoon fine sea salt

½ teaspoon ground black pepper

1. In a large saucepan, over medium-low heat, bring stock to simmer. Drop okra in stock, stirring slowly and frequently, until slightly softened, about 4 minutes. Remove from stock and place on a work surface, reserving stock in the saucepan.

2. Push peppercorns into the center of okra. Return to broth; add butter or ghee, cumin, salt, and pepper. Serve warm.

Per Serving Calories: 33 | Fat: 3g | Protein: 1g | Sodium: 578mg | Fiber: 1.5g | Carbohydrates: 3g | Sugar: 0.5g

Jicama "Rice"

You can make "rice" out of jicama, just as you can out of cauliflower! Jicama are slightly sweeter and a bit starchier than cauliflower. The knobby white root is low in calories and high in fiber and antioxidants. It's also a good source of vitamins C and B, in addition to magnesium, copper, and iron.

PREP TIME: 10 MINUTES
COOK TIME: 10–12 MINUTES

INGREDIENTS | SERVES 4

1 large jicama
1 tablespoon lemon juice
2 tablespoons coconut oil
2 medium shallots, peeled and minced
½ teaspoon fine sea salt
⅛ teaspoon ground white pepper

1. Peel jicama and grate with a box grater or in a food processor. Sprinkle with lemon juice and mix.

2. In large skillet, melt coconut oil over medium heat. Add shallots; cook and stir until tender, about 4 minutes.

3. Add grated jicama to skillet; cook and stir until jicama releases some of its water and the water evaporates, about 5–6 minutes. Taste jicama to see if it's tender. If not, cook another 1–2 minutes. Sprinkle with salt and pepper and serve.

Per Serving Calories: 179 | Fat: 7g | Protein: 3g | Sodium: 304mg | Fiber: 13g | Carbohydrates: 28g | Sugar: 8g

Moroccan Root Vegetables

Root vegetables are flavored with Moroccan spices for a twist on an everyday favorite.

PREP TIME: 15 MINUTES
COOK TIME: 9 HOURS

INGREDIENTS | SERVES 8

1 pound parsnips, peeled and diced

1 pound turnips, peeled and diced

2 medium onions, peeled and chopped

1 pound carrots, peeled and diced

6 dried apricots, chopped

4 pitted prunes, chopped

1 teaspoon ground turmeric

1 teaspoon ground cumin

½ teaspoon ground ginger

½ teaspoon ground cinnamon

¼ teaspoon ground cayenne pepper

1 tablespoon dried parsley

1 tablespoon dried cilantro

14 ounces Basic Vegetable Stock (see recipe in Chapter 6)

Add all ingredients to a 4- or 6-quart slow cooker. Cover and cook on low 9 hours or until vegetables are cooked through. Drain liquid and serve warm.

Per Serving   Calories: 107 | Fat: 0.5g | Protein: 2g | Sodium: 82mg | Fiber: 6g | Carbohydrates: 26g | Sugar: 11.5g

Cauliflower "Rice"

Cauliflower makes a surprisingly delicious substitute for rice. Just be sure you don't overcook it. You want each little piece of cauliflower to be tender, but slightly firm to stand up to the sauces and foods you'll serve with it.

PREP TIME: 10 MINUTES
COOK TIME: 9–10 MINUTES

INGREDIENTS | SERVES 4

1 large head cauliflower, florets separated

1 tablespoon lemon juice

2 tablespoons coconut oil

3 small shallots, peeled and minced

2 cloves garlic, peeled and minced

1 teaspoon fine sea salt

⅛ teaspoon ground white pepper

1. Using a box grater or a food processer, grate or process florets into tiny pieces. Toss with lemon juice and set aside.

2. In a large skillet, melt coconut oil over medium-high heat. Add shallots and garlic; cook and stir until tender, about 5 minutes.

3. Add cauliflower and sprinkle with salt and pepper. Cook 4–5 minutes, stirring frequently, until cauliflower is tender but somewhat firm in the center. Serve immediately.

Per Serving   Calories: 121 | Fat 7g | Protein: 5g | Sodium: 660mg | Fiber: 6g | Carbohydrates: 13g | Sugar: 4g

Cajun Collard Greens

Like Brussels sprouts and kimchi, collard greens are one of those foods folks tend to either love or hate. They're highly nutritious, so hopefully this recipe will turn you into a collards lover, if you're not already.

PREP TIME: 5 MINUTES
COOK TIME: 30 MINUTES

INGREDIENTS | SERVES 4

2 tablespoons olive oil

1 medium onion, peeled and diced

3 cloves garlic, peeled and minced

1 pound collard greens, chopped

¾ cup water or Basic Vegetable Stock (see recipe in Chapter 6)

1 (14-ounce) can no-salt-added diced tomatoes, drained

1½ teaspoons Cajun seasoning

½ teaspoon hot sauce

¼ teaspoon sea salt

1. In a large skillet, heat oil over medium heat. Add onion, garlic, and collard greens and sauté 3–5 minutes until onion is soft.

2. Add water or stock, tomatoes, and Cajun seasoning. Bring to a simmer over low heat, cover, and cook 20 minutes or until greens are soft, stirring occasionally.

3. Remove lid, stir in hot sauce and salt, and cook uncovered another 1–2 minutes to allow excess moisture to evaporate.

Per Serving   Calories: 121 | Fat: 7g | Protein: 5g | Sodium: 660mg | Fiber: 6g | Carbohydrates: 13g | Sugar: 4g

Baked Stuffed Artichokes

These are worth a bit of effort. You can prepare them in advance, then finish cooking just before serving.

PREP TIME: 15 MINUTES
COOK TIME: 1 HOUR

INGREDIENTS | SERVES 4

2 large artichokes

2 tablespoons avocado oil

2 cloves garlic, peeled and chopped

½ sweet onion, peeled and chopped

1 cup almond meal

1 tablespoon minced lemon peel

8 raw medium shrimp, peeled and deveined

¼ cup chopped fresh parsley

½ teaspoon ground black pepper

4 quarts plus ½ cup water

Juice and rind of ½ large lemon

½ teaspoon ground coriander

1. Remove any tough or brown outside leaves from artichokes. Using a sharp knife, cut off artichoke tops about ½" down. Slam artichokes against a countertop to loosen leaves. Cut in half, from top to stem, and set aside.

2. Heat oil in a large frying pan over medium heat. Add garlic and onion and sauté 5 minutes, stirring. Add almond meal, lemon peel, shrimp, parsley, and pepper. Cook until shrimp turns pink. Pulse shrimp mixture in a food processor or blender.

3. In a large stockpot bring 4 quarts water to a boil. Add artichokes, lemon juice, lemon rind, and coriander and boil 18 minutes. Remove artichokes and reserve cooking water.

4. Place artichokes in a baking dish with ½ cup water in the bottom. Pile with shrimp filling. Drizzle with a bit of the cooking water and bake 25 minutes. Serve.

Per Serving Calories: 256 | Fat: 18g | Protein: 4g | Sodium: 171mg | Fiber: 7g | Carbohydrates: 17.5g | Sugar: 3g

Deviled Eggs

Eggs are a staple in the Paleo diet. This is a quick recipe that can be whipped up in no time. Kids and adults will love these, and they can be easily served at parties or family gatherings.

PREP TIME: 45 MINUTES
COOK TIME: N/A

INGREDIENTS | SERVES 10

10 large hard-boiled eggs

3 tablespoons Homemade Mayonnaise (see recipe in Chapter 16)

2 green onions, finely chopped

2 cloves garlic, peeled and finely chopped

1 large stalk celery, finely chopped

1 teaspoon dry mustard

1/8 teaspoon sea salt

1 teaspoon ground black pepper

1/4 teaspoon sweet paprika

1. Peel eggs, cut in half lengthwise, and separate yolks from whites.

2. Combine egg yolks, mayonnaise, onions, garlic, celery, mustard, salt, and pepper. Mix well to form paste.

3. Stuff egg whites with yolk mixture.

4. Sprinkle paprika over eggs and chill for at least 30 minutes before serving. Keep in refrigerator for up to 2 days.

Per Serving Calories: 119 | Fat: 8.5g | Protein: 6.5g | Sodium: 97mg | Fiber: 0.3g | Carbohydrates: 1g | Sugar: 1g

CHAPTER 14

Baked Goods and Desserts

Paleo Sandwich Bread

This basic bread recipe allows you to carry on life as usual if you're used to eating toast or sandwiches. Bake it in large batches, slice, and freeze for quick and easy access.

PREP TIME: 1 HOUR
COOK TIME: 50–60 MINUTES

INGREDIENTS | SERVES 10

Coconut oil, for greasing pan
4 large eggs, yolks separated from whites
1 cup unsweetened almond butter
2 tablespoons Grade B maple syrup
3 tablespoons unsweetened applesauce
1 tablespoon lemon juice
¼ cup unsweetened almond milk
¼ cup coconut flour
1 teaspoon baking soda
½ teaspoon cream of tartar
½ teaspoon fine sea salt
¼ teaspoon vanilla extract

Nut Butter Swaps

You can use any Paleo nut butter for this recipe to get slightly different flavor combinations. You can even make your own nut butter by using a food processor to grind nuts into a creamy paste.

1. Preheat oven to 300°F. Grease an 8" × 4" loaf pan with coconut oil.

2. In a small mixing bowl, whip egg whites with a whisk until they form soft peaks. In a separate medium mixing bowl, combine all other ingredients and stir by hand or with a mixer until thoroughly mixed.

3. Add egg whites to batter and lightly stir until just combined. Don't overmix.

4. Pour batter into prepared pan and place in the oven. Bake 50–60 minutes or until the center of the bread passes the toothpick test (if the toothpick comes out clean, the bread is ready).

5. Remove from oven and let cool. Slice and serve, or freeze for later use. Store in refrigerator 5 days or in freezer 6 months.

Per Serving (1 slice) Calories: 213 | Fat: 16g | Protein: 9g | Sodium: 356mg | Fiber: 4g | Carbohydrates: 11g | Sugar: 4g

Ginger Lemon Muffins

These zesty muffins are a perfect complement to your morning coffee, or served as a dessert when topped with Creamy Vanilla Frosting (see recipe in this chapter).

PREP TIME: 25 MINUTES
COOK TIME: 15–17 MINUTES

INGREDIENTS | SERVES 12

½ cup ghee
½ cup coconut sugar
¼ cup raw honey
2 large eggs
1 tablespoon ground ginger
2 tablespoons lemon zest
1 cup almond flour
1 cup cassava flour
½ teaspoon baking soda
½ teaspoon cream of tartar
1 cup full-fat coconut milk

1. Preheat oven to 375°F. Line a muffin pan with parchment liners.

2. In a small mixing bowl whip together ghee, sugar, honey, and eggs until creamy. Stir in remaining ingredients until thoroughly mixed.

3. Fill muffin cups about ¾ full and bake 15–17 minutes or until they pass the toothpick test (if the toothpick comes out clean, the muffins are ready). Let cool 10 minutes before serving. Store in refrigerator up to 5 days or in freezer up to 6 months.

Per Serving Calories: 277 | Fat: 19g | Protein: 2g | Sodium: 66mg | Fiber: 2g | Carbohydrates: 26.5g | Sugar: 14g

What on Earth Is a Cassava?

Cassava flour is made from yuca (also known as cassava), a root vegetable that is similar to parsnips and turnips. It is a starchy white flour that is Paleo-friendly because it's completely grain-free.

Almond Apple Muffins

These muffins are comforting thanks to the familiar warmth of cinnamon, and super moist because of the applesauce! Whether warm or cold, these muffins are sure to be a hit.

PREP TIME: 25 MINUTES
COOK TIME: 25–30 MINUTES

INGREDIENTS | SERVES 12

1 large Granny Smith apple, peeled, cored, and diced

½ cup unsweetened applesauce

3 tablespoons raw honey

1 cup almond flour

½ cup cassava flour, or more as necessary

2 large eggs

3 tablespoons ghee

1 tablespoon ground cinnamon

½ teaspoon baking soda

¼ teaspoon cream of tartar

⅛ teaspoon fine sea salt

1. Preheat oven to 350°F. Line a muffin pan with parchment liners.

2. In a large mixing bowl, combine all ingredients and stir thoroughly. Batter should be somewhat thick. If the batter seems too soupy, add more cassava flour (about ¼ cup).

3. Evenly fill muffin cups and bake 25–30 minutes or until they pass the toothpick test (if the toothpick comes out clean, the muffins are ready). Remove from oven and let cool 10 minutes.

Per Serving   Calories: 142 | Fat: 8g | Protein: 1g | Sodium: 87mg | Fiber: 2g | Carbohydrates: 15.5g | Sugar: 7g

Banana-Coconut Bread

This banana-coconut loaf recipe can double as a dessert recipe quite nicely.
Serve with fresh banana and strawberry slices for a completely yummy treat.

PREP TIME: 40 MINUTES
COOK TIME: 45 MINUTES

INGREDIENTS | SERVES 8

1¼ cups almond meal
2 teaspoons baking powder
¼ teaspoon baking soda
½ cup strawberry purée
¼ teaspoon ground cinnamon
2 large eggs
3 large ripe bananas, mashed
¼ cup flaxseed flour
½ cup chopped walnuts
1 cup unsweetened coconut flakes

1. Preheat oven to 350°F. Grease a 9" × 5" loaf pan with coconut oil.

2. Combine almond meal, baking powder, baking soda, strawberry purée, cinnamon, eggs, bananas, and flour in a large bowl. Mix well.

3. Fold chopped walnuts and coconut flakes into batter (do not overmix). Pour batter into prepared pan.

4. Bake 45 minutes or until a wooden toothpick inserted into the center of the loaf comes out dry.

5. Let cool 5 minutes, then transfer to a wire rack to cool completely.

Per Serving Calories: 274 | Fat: 19g | Protein: 5g | Sodium: 182mg | Fiber: 6g | Carbohydrates: 22g | Sugar: 8g

Fruit Purées

Fruit purées are a great way to add sweetness to any recipe. Simply place your favorite fruit in a food processor and quickly pulse to chop finely. Use in place of syrups and jams.

Chocolate Pudding

This pudding tastes so decadent that no one will ever know
there are healthy fats and superfoods hidden within.

PREP TIME: 30 MINUTES
COOK TIME: N/A

INGREDIENTS | SERVES 2

1 large ripe banana, frozen

2 pitted dates

2 tablespoons raw cacao powder

1 large ripe avocado, peeled and pitted

1 cup full-fat coconut milk

½ teaspoon vanilla extract

1 teaspoon Grade B maple syrup

2 tablespoons raw honey

½ tablespoon matcha powder

½ tablespoon chlorella powder

Combine all ingredients in a food processor and pulse until creamy and smooth. Chill in refrigerator before serving.

Per Serving Calories: 558 | Fat: 33g | Protein: 6g | Sodium: 20mg | Fiber: 9g | Carbohydrates: 65g | Sugar: 44g

Caramel Walnut Glazed Apples

This warm and sweet dessert is perfect on its own or as a topping
for bread, granola, or even ice cream (as long as it's Paleo, of course!).

PREP TIME: 5 MINUTES
COOK TIME: 17–20 MINUTES

INGREDIENTS | SERVES 6

¼ cup slivered walnuts

⅓ cup coconut sugar

2 tablespoons ghee

1 teaspoon vanilla extract

1 teaspoon ground cinnamon

1 large Granny Smith apple, cored and cut into ½" slices

1 large Honeycrisp apple, cored and cut into ½" slices

1. In a large skillet over medium heat, toast walnuts until lightly browned, about 5 minutes. Remove walnuts from pan and set aside.

2. In the same skillet, combine sugar, ghee, vanilla, and cinnamon over medium heat, stirring frequently until sugar is dissolved and mixture starts to thicken, about 5 minutes. Add apples and continue to cook over medium heat, stirring often, 7–10 minutes until apples soften.

3. Remove from heat, stir in walnuts, and serve warm.

Per Serving Calories: 158 | Fat: 8g | Protein: 1g | Sodium: 2mg | Fiber: 2g | Carbohydrates: 21.5g | Sugar: 18g

Honey Spiced Pumpkin

*This sweet dessert mimics the flavor of pumpkin pie,
but without the crust and with an exceptionally easy prep!*

PREP TIME: 1 HOUR 5 MINUTES
COOK TIME: N/A

INGREDIENTS | SERVES 4

1 (15-ounce) can pumpkin purée

½ cup full-fat coconut milk

2 tablespoons raw honey

1 tablespoon Grade B maple syrup

½ teaspoon ground cinnamon

¼ teaspoon ground nutmeg

⅛ teaspoon ground allspice

⅛ teaspoon ground ginger

1 teaspoon vanilla extract

Combine all ingredients in a food processor or in a medium mixing bowl using a hand mixer. Chill at least 1 hour before serving. Keep in refrigerator up to 3 days.

Per Serving Calories: 123 | Fat: 6g | Protein: 2g | Sodium: 6mg | Fiber: 3g | Carbohydrates: 17g | Sugar: 13.5g

Creamy Vanilla Frosting

*This frosting is perfect paired with the Paleo Carrot Spice Cake
(see recipe in this chapter), but can also be used to frost any dessert.*

PREP TIME: 5 MINUTES
COOK TIME: N/A

INGREDIENTS | SERVES 12

½ cup coconut butter

¼ cup raw honey

1 cup raw cacao nibs

1 teaspoon vanilla extract

½ teaspoon ground cinnamon

Blend together all ingredients in a medium bowl and whisk thoroughly. Refrigerate for up to 3 days.

Per Serving Calories: 176 | Fat: 12g | Protein: 1g | Sodium: 2mg | Fiber: 3g | Carbohydrates: 6g | Sugar: 6g

Paleo Carrot Spice Cake

This carrot cake is sweet and spicy just like the traditional version, and thanks to the carrots and applesauce, it is super moist. Topped with Creamy Vanilla Frosting, this cake is sure to become a Paleo favorite for birthdays, holidays, and just-because-you-need-cake days.

PREP TIME: 1 HOUR 25 MINUTES
COOK TIME: 30–35 MINUTES

INGREDIENTS | SERVES 12

Coconut oil, for greasing pan
¾ cup coconut sugar
¾ cup raw honey
¾ cup ghee
3 large eggs
1½ cups almond flour
½ cup cassava flour
1 tablespoon ground cinnamon
1 teaspoon baking soda
1 teaspoon cream of tartar
2 teaspoons vanilla extract
½ teaspoon fine sea salt
6 medium carrots, peeled and shredded (about 3 cups packed)
½ cup unsweetened applesauce
1 recipe Creamy Vanilla Frosting (see recipe in this chapter)

1. Preheat oven to 350°F. Grease a 9" × 13" cake pan with coconut oil.

2. In a large mixing bowl, combine sugar, honey, ghee, and eggs with a hand mixer or by hand until thoroughly mixed. Add flours, cinnamon, baking soda, cream of tartar, vanilla, and salt and continue mixing until blended, about 1 minute.

3. Stir carrots and applesauce into mixture by hand until carrots are well coated. Pour into prepared pan and level the top.

4. Bake 30–35 minutes or until the center passes the toothpick test (if the toothpick comes out clean, the cake is ready). Remove from heat and let cool at least 1 hour before frosting.

Per Serving   Calories: 556 | Fat: 35g | Protein: 3g | Sodium: 243mg | Fiber: 6g | Carbohydrates: 55g | Sugar: 39g

Chia Fudge Brownies

When you need a chocolate fix, these fudgy brownies will come to your rescue. Packed with super-hydrating chia seeds, these brownies will be moist, chewy, and absolutely satisfying.

PREP TIME: 13–17 HOURS
COOK TIME: 20–25 MINUTES

INGREDIENTS | SERVES 12

½ cup water
1 tablespoon whole chia seeds
Coconut oil, for greasing pan
½ cup raw cacao powder
½ cup cashew butter
¼ teaspoon baking soda
1 cup coconut sugar
2 large eggs
1 teaspoon vanilla extract

1. Combine water and chia seeds in a small bowl. Cover and let stand 12–16 hours. Stir.

2. Grease a 9" × 9" baking pan with coconut oil. Preheat oven to 350°F.

3. In a mixing bowl, combine soaked chia seeds with remaining ingredients, stirring thoroughly by hand or with a hand mixer.

4. Spread mixture into prepared pan and bake 20–25 minutes or until the center passes the toothpick test (if the toothpick comes out clean, the fudge is ready). Let cool and then cut into 12 squares.

Per Serving Calories: 158 | Fat: 7g | Protein: 4g | Sodium: 39mg | Fiber: 1g | Carbohydrates: 22g | Sugar: 17g

Mocha Bites

This recipe will satisfy your chocolate craving while giving you a hint of roasted coffee flavor, making these a decadent dessert that packs an antioxidant-rich punch.

PREP TIME: 1 HOUR 10 MINUTES
COOK TIME: N/A

INGREDIENTS | SERVES 18

1½ cups raw cashews

1½ cups walnuts

2 teaspoons fine sea salt

1 tablespoon vanilla extract

2 cups pitted dates

⅓ cup water

⅔ cup raw cacao powder

2 tablespoons finely ground dark roast coffee

1. Combine nuts and salt in a food processor and pulse until finely chopped. Do not overpulse or nuts will turn into nut butter.

2. Add vanilla, dates, and water and pulse until mixture is combined.

3. Add cacao and coffee and pulse to combine.

4. Shape mixture into 18 equal-sized balls (about 1"). Refrigerate 1 hour to set in a covered bowl. Serve chilled. Keep in refrigerator up to 4 days.

Per Serving (1 ball)   Calories: 198 | Fat: 12g | Protein: 5g | Sodium: 251mg | Fiber: 3g | Carbohydrates: 20g | Sugar: 11g

Any Nuts Will Do

This recipe works well with any type of nut, so use what you have on hand or experiment with different blends. Try hazelnuts, pecans, Brazil nuts, and even sunflower seeds for slightly different flavor and nutrient profiles.

Cashew Cookies

*These cookies are soft and chewy just like non-Paleo cookies,
and they taste delicious when dipped in almond milk or coconut cream.*

PREP TIME: 20 MINUTES
COOK TIME: 15–20 MINUTES

INGREDIENTS | SERVES 12

1 cup cashew butter
1 large egg
1 teaspoon baking soda
½ cup coconut sugar
½ cup raw cacao powder
1 teaspoon vanilla extract
1 teaspoon ghee

1. Preheat oven to 350°F. Line a cookie sheet with parchment paper.

2. In a large mixing bowl, combine all ingredients until thoroughly mixed. Alternately, combine all ingredients in a food processor until the mixture is completely smooth.

3. Spoon out mixture onto cookie sheet in 12 equal portions. Use a fork to flatten dough into round cookies. Bake 15–20 minutes or until golden brown. Remove from oven and allow to cool 10 minutes before removing from cookie sheet.

Per Serving (1 cookie) Calories: 180 | Fat: 11g | Protein: 5g | Sodium: 113mg | Fiber: 1g | Carbohydrates: 16g | Sugar: 8g

Paleo Chocolate Bars

Your kids will be thrilled when they see these chocolate bars in their lunchboxes. These bars are quick to whip up and quick to eat. The amount of honey can be varied depending on your desired sweetness level.

PREP TIME: 20 MINUTES–1 HOUR 10 MINUTES
COOK TIME: 3–5 MINUTES

INGREDIENTS | SERVES 8

1 tablespoon raw honey
¼ cup coconut oil
¼ cup ground almonds
¼ cup ground hazelnuts
¼ cup sunflower seeds
¼ cup raw cacao powder
¾ cup unsweetened coconut flakes

1. Melt honey and coconut oil in a small saucepan over medium heat.

2. In a medium mixing bowl, combine almonds, hazelnuts, sunflower seeds, cacao powder, and coconut. Mix thoroughly.

3. Add honey mixture to bowl and mix well.

4. Pour mixture into an 8" × 8" baking pan lined with parchment paper and freeze about 10 minutes or refrigerate about 1 hour.

5. Cut into squares and enjoy.

Per Serving Calories: 184 | Fat: 16.5g | Protein: 3g | Sodium: 1mg | Fiber: 2.5g | Carbohydrates: 8g | Sugar: 3g

Natural Sugars

Although natural honey is an acceptable Paleolithic diet food, you should still eat it in moderation. It does cause an increase in blood sugar levels and therefore a spike in insulin.

Blueberry Cookie Balls

These antioxidant-packed cookie balls are a great alternative to commercial cookies.
They taste great, are all natural, and will give your kids energy from all macronutrient categories.

PREP TIME: 1 HOUR 40 MINUTES
COOK TIME: 12–15 MINUTES

INGREDIENTS | SERVES 12

2 large egg whites

5 cups blueberries

3 teaspoons ground cinnamon

1½ teaspoons ground ginger

¼ cup raw honey

1 teaspoon vanilla extract

Glycemic Load and Autoimmunity

It is particularly important to limit sugar intake when trying to heal from thyroid disease, because the body is more sensitive to mood changes and inflammation that result from unstable blood sugar. Recipes that combine fat, protein, and carbohydrates minimize blood sugar spikes and pitfalls.

1. Preheat oven to 350°F.

2. Whisk egg whites in a large bowl until frothy. Add all other ingredients and mix well.

3. Scoop out tablespoons of dough and form into 12 balls. Place balls on a parchment-lined baking sheet. Bake 12–15 minutes.

4. Transfer cookies to a wire rack to cool. When cookies are completely cool, place in a single layer on a clean baking sheet and refrigerate 1 hour before serving.

Per Serving (1 ball) Calories: 62 | Fat: 0.1g | Protein: 1g | Sodium: 9mg | Fiber: 2g | Carbohydrates: 15g | Sugar: 12g

CHAPTER 15

Smoothies and Drinks

Spiced Coconut Coffee

This spiced beverage is perfect for special occasions, holidays, or a satisfying cup of comfort in the morning.

PREP TIME: 5 MINUTES
COOK TIME: 15 MINUTES

INGREDIENTS | SERVES 4

¼ cup slivered almonds

4 cups water

1 tablespoon ground cinnamon

1 teaspoon ground nutmeg

¼ cup coconut sugar

⅓ cup coarsely ground dark roast coffee

Cut the Caffeine

Even if you're avoiding caffeine or want to enjoy this beverage later in the day, you can still enjoy this spiced coffee drink by using decaf coffee. Don't like coffee? Make the recipe using loose-leaf black tea.

1. In a medium saucepan over medium heat, toast almonds until lightly browned, about 2–3 minutes.

2. Add water, cinnamon, nutmeg, and sugar to saucepan and bring to a boil. Reduce heat to medium-low and simmer 3 minutes.

3. Remove saucepan from heat and immediately stir in coffee. Let steep 5 minutes, and then strain through a coffee filter, cheesecloth, or fine metal sieve. Serve warm or over ice.

Per Serving Calories: 71 | Fat: 0.4g | Protein: 1g | Sodium: 10mg | Fiber: 1g | Carbohydrates: 18g | Sugar: 13g

Hot Almond Cream

This coffee-less beverage has all the warmth and comfort of a latte without any dairy or caffeine. Serve it for brunch or a post-dinner dessert.

PREP TIME: 5 MINUTES
COOK TIME: 5 MINUTES

INGREDIENTS | SERVES 4

¼ cup ghee
¼ cup coconut sugar
¼ cup raw honey
1 cup full-fat coconut milk
1 cup unsweetened almond milk
½ teaspoon almond extract
½ teaspoon vanilla extract

In a medium saucepan over medium heat combine all ingredients. Simmer 5 minutes, stirring frequently. Remove from heat and serve warm. For a festive appearance, sprinkle with a bit of ground cinnamon or top with coconut whipped cream.

Per Serving Calories: 367 | Fat: 27g | Protein: 1.5g | Sodium: 47mg | Fiber: 0g | Carbohydrates: 31g | Sugar: 30g

Choosing Almond Milk Brands

If you search the shelves in the grocery store, you'll find numerous brands. The key to selecting a good premade almond milk is to choose one that is unsweetened and one that does not contain inflammatory ingredients such as carrageenan or anything else that is distinctly not Paleo. Simple Truth Unsweetened Almondmilk is a good option, along with Silk Unsweetened Almondmilk.

Paleo Chai Latte

This warm and soothing classic beverage is paleoized here with the use of coconut milk. Try experimenting for a personalized flavor by slightly altering spice amounts to your taste preference.

PREP TIME: 2 MINUTES
COOK TIME: 5 MINUTES

INGREDIENTS | SERVES 1

1½ cups full-fat coconut milk
¼ teaspoon ground cardamom
½ teaspoon ground cinnamon
¼ teaspoon ground ginger
¼ teaspoon ground nutmeg
⅛ teaspoon ground cloves
¼ teaspoon vanilla extract

In a small saucepan, combine all ingredients over medium heat. Simmer 5 minutes or until hot.

Per Serving Calories: 677 | Fat: 68g | Protein: 7g | Sodium: 44mg | Fiber: 1g | Carbohydrates: 12g | Sugar: 0.2g

Apple Carrot Smoothie

This smoothie takes the complementary flavors of apples and carrots and combines them with plant-based protein to create an antioxidant-rich meal-replacement beverage.

PREP TIME: 5 MINUTES
COOK TIME: N/A

INGREDIENTS | SERVES 1

1 large carrot, peeled and chopped
1 medium apple, cored and sliced
1 cup water
1 cup coconut water
1 tablespoon hemp protein powder
½ tablespoon pumpkin seeds
1 packed cup chard
2 teaspoons raw honey

Combine all ingredients in a blender, food processor, or NutriBullet and pulse until well combined and smooth. Serve chilled.

Per Serving Calories: 249 | Fat: 3g | Protein: 7g | Sodium: 197mg | Fiber: 7g | Carbohydrates: 54g | Sugar: 41g

Paleo Cappuccino

This creamy coffee beverage is rich in good-for-you fats,
making it a frothy and filling beverage that can actually double as your breakfast.

PREP TIME: 5 MINUTES
COOK TIME: 5 MINUTES
INGREDIENTS | SERVES 1

8 ounces brewed coffee

1 tablespoon ghee

½ tablespoon coconut oil

¼ cup coconut cream

1 teaspoon collagen powder

1 tablespoon raw honey

2 teaspoons vanilla extract

In a small saucepan over medium heat, combine all ingredients and simmer 5 minutes or until hot. Remove from heat and whisk by hand or pulse in a blender or food processor until frothy. Serve warm.

Per Serving   Calories: 411 | Fat: 33g | Protein: 2g | Sodium: 20mg | Fiber: 0g | Carbohydrates: 20g | Sugar: 20g

Why Raw Honey?

Raw honey is superior to refined forms of honey because it still contains antioxidants, unlike its cooked counterpart. As with any Paleo food, unprocessed versions are always preferred over ingredients that are highly processed.

Chocolate Coffee Smoothie

This rich, chocolaty smoothie can hold its own against any dessert, but is also the perfect snack or meal-replacement beverage. Top with raw cacao nibs for an extra treat.

PREP TIME: 5 MINUTES

COOK TIME: N/A

INGREDIENTS | SERVES 1

1 cup brewed coffee, chilled

1 cup full-fat coconut milk, chilled

1 small avocado, pitted and peeled

2 tablespoons raw cacao powder

1 tablespoon unsweetened almond butter

1 teaspoon vanilla extract

1 tablespoon raw honey

Combine all ingredients in a blender, food processor, or NutriBullet and pulse until well combined and smooth. Serve chilled.

Per Serving   Calories: 880 | Fat: 73g | Protein: 13g | Sodium: 93mg | Fiber: 13g | Carbohydrates: 45g | Sugar: 18g

Avocado in My Coffee?

Avocado is such a versatile fruit; when combined with stronger flavors such as chocolate and coffee, it blends with the predominant flavors and can go completely undetected. In this smoothie it lends a nice dose of healthy fat and makes the smoothie rich and filling.

Fruit and Spinach Smoothie

If you're not a fan of leafy green vegetables, get them down by disguising them with the prevailing flavors of pineapples, apples, and oranges.

PREP TIME: 5 MINUTES
COOK TIME: N/A

INGREDIENTS | SERVES 1

1 packed cup spinach
½ cup pineapple chunks
½ cup unsweetened pineapple juice
Juice of 1 medium orange
1 small apple, cored and sliced
1 cup unsweetened coconut water

Combine all ingredients in a blender, food processor, or NutriBullet and pulse until well combined and smooth. Serve chilled.

Per Serving Calories: 247 | Fat: 0.3g | Protein: 3g | Sodium: 88mg | Fiber: 4g | Carbohydrates: 62g | Sugar: 49g

Folate for Fertility

Even if you're not trying to have a baby, a healthy body is a fertile body. Folate, an essential B vitamin, is found in abundance in leafy greens and is well absorbed when consumed in this way. Two cups of spinach contain more than 100 percent of the recommended daily amount.

Peach and Kiwi Protein Smoothie

This smoothie is perfect for a meal on the go or as a standalone breakfast.

PREP TIME: 5 MINUTES
COOK TIME: N/A

INGREDIENTS | SERVES 1

1 small kiwifruit, peeled and sliced

1 packed cup spinach

1 small peach, pitted and sliced

1 small ripe avocado, pitted and peeled

1½ tablespoons hemp protein powder

1½ cups unsweetened coconut water

1 large orange, juiced

1 cup ice chips

2 teaspoons raw honey

Combine all ingredients in a blender, food processor, or NutriBullet and pulse until well combined and smooth. Serve chilled.

Per Serving Calories: 509 | Fat: 20.5g | Protein: 12g | Sodium: 130mg | Fiber: 17g | Carbohydrates: 73.5g | Sugar: 50g

Tropical Cream Smoothie

This ultra-smooth beverage will make you feel like you're drinking up dessert while kicking back on a Hawaiian vacation.

PREP TIME: 5 MINUTES
COOK TIME: N/A

INGREDIENTS | SERVES 1

½ cup pineapple chunks

½ cup unsweetened pineapple juice

½ cup coconut cream

½ cup unsweetened coconut water

½ cup ice chips

1 tablespoon coconut nectar

Combine all ingredients in a blender, food processor, or NutriBullet and pulse until well combined and smooth. Serve chilled.

Per Serving Calories: 424 | Fat: 24g | Protein: 1g | Sodium: 73mg | Fiber: 1g | Carbohydrates: 49g | Sugar: 42g

Ginger Green Smoothie

This green drink is rich in antioxidants and vitamins and is the perfect addition to a protein-heavy breakfast or a great post-workout recovery drink.

PREP TIME: 5 MINUTES
COOK TIME: N/A

INGREDIENTS | SERVES 1

1 packed cup chard

1 small apple, peeled, cored, and sliced

2 slices pickled ginger

2 teaspoons raw honey

1 cup water, or more as needed

Combine all ingredients in a blender, food processor, or NutriBullet and pulse until well combined and smooth. Add more water as needed to reach desired consistency. Serve chilled.

Per Serving Calories: 121 | Fat: 0.1g | Protein: 1g | Sodium: 245mg | Fiber: 3g | Carbohydrates: 30.5g | Sugar: 25g

Give It More Ginger

Replace the water in this recipe with brewed ginger tea for an extra boost to your digestive system. Ginger tea is also great at soothing stomach nausea, so the next time you get a stomach bug, make this your go-to. Not only will it settle your stomach, but it's packed with nutrients that will help your body recover faster.

Cleansing Green Smoothie

Boost your liver's ability to remove harmful toxins from your body by drinking this cleansing smoothie first thing in the morning as a precursor to breakfast.

PREP TIME: 5 MINUTES
COOK TIME: N/A

INGREDIENTS | SERVES 1

¼ cup dandelion greens
¼ cup beet greens
½ cup baby spinach
½ cup chard
1 small pear, cored and quartered
1 small ripe banana, peeled
1½ cups unsweetened coconut water
2 teaspoons raw honey

Combine all ingredients in a blender, food processor, or NutriBullet until well combined and smooth. Serve chilled. May be stored in refrigerator up to 1 day.

Per Serving   Calories: 392 | Fat: 0.4g | Protein: 4g | Sodium: 177mg | Fiber: 9g | Carbohydrates: 98g | Sugar: 76g

Let It Out

Dandelion greens and other dark leafy greens are rich in nutrients that help the liver complete both phases of detox. Phase 1 involves collecting and compacting toxins from the bloodstream, while Phase 2 involves combining with water-soluble molecules for elimination from the body via the kidneys and intestines.

Super Berry Protein Smoothie

This protein-packed smoothie is rich with flavors of berries and greens, and naturally sweetened with dates and honey, making it the perfect on-the-go breakfast or snack.

PREP TIME: 5 MINUTES
COOK TIME: N/A

INGREDIENTS | SERVES 1

1 large ripe banana, peeled
½ cup blueberries
½ cup strawberries
1½ cups full-fat coconut milk
1 tablespoon hemp protein powder
1 tablespoon collagen powder
½ cup baby spinach
2 teaspoons raw honey
2 pitted dates

Combine all ingredients in a blender, food processor, or NutriBullet and pulse until well combined and smooth. Serve chilled.

Per Serving Calories: 1,085 | Fat: 69g | Protein: 20g | Sodium: 76mg | Fiber: 12g | Carbohydrates: 107g | Sugar: 71g

Mango Berry Smoothie

Watercress acts as a mild background green for this deliciously sweet and smooth recipe. The mangoes, raspberries, and coconut milk provide a healthy serving of vitamins, minerals, and antioxidants.

PREP TIME: 5 MINUTES
COOK TIME: N/A

INGREDIENTS | SERVES 4

1 cup chopped watercress
2 medium mangoes, pitted and peeled
2 pints raspberries
1½ cups full-fat coconut milk, divided

1. Place watercress, mangoes, raspberries, and ¾ cup coconut milk in a blender and blend until thoroughly combined.

2. Add remaining coconut milk while blending until desired consistency is achieved.

Per Serving Calories: 332 | Fat: 18g | Protein: 5g | Sodium: 16mg | Fiber: 11g | Carbohydrates: 42g | Sugar: 28g

Mangoes and Digestion

Mangoes aid in digestion by combating uncomfortable acids in the digestive system and creating a more balanced system capable of a smooth, regular digestive process.

Cucumber-Mint Smoothie

The light taste of cucumber and fragrant mint combine with deep green romaine in this refreshing smoothie.

PREP TIME: 5 MINUTES
COOK TIME: N/A

INGREDIENTS | SERVES 4

1 cup chopped romaine lettuce

2 medium cucumbers, peeled and quartered

¼ cup chopped fresh mint

1 cup water, divided

1. Place romaine, cucumbers, mint, and ½ cup water in a blender and combine thoroughly.

2. Add remaining water while blending until desired consistency is achieved. Chill before serving or serve immediately.

Per Serving Calories: 14 | Fat: 0.1g | Protein: 1g | Sodium: 5mg | Fiber: 1g | Carbohydrates: 3g | Sugar: 1.5g

Cucumbers Aren't Just Water

Even though a cucumber is mostly water (and fiber), it is far more than a tasty, hydrating, and filling snack option. These green vegetables are a great addition to your diet, especially if your skin is in need of moisture and clarity! A clear complexion is an aesthetic benefit of consuming cucumbers.

Sweet and Savory Beet Smoothie

Beets and their greens are filled with antioxidants and vitamins. Paired with flavorful carrots and cucumbers, they create a sweet and healthy smoothie you're sure to enjoy.

PREP TIME: 5 MINUTES
COOK TIME: N/A

INGREDIENTS | SERVES 4

1 cup chopped beet greens
2 medium beets, peeled and chopped
2 medium carrots, peeled and chopped
1 medium cucumber, peeled and chopped
2 cups water, divided

1. Place beet greens, beets, carrots, cucumber, and 1 cup water in a blender and blend until thoroughly combined.

2. Add remaining 1 cup water while blending until desired consistency is achieved. Serve immediately or chill for up to 2 hours before serving.

Per Serving   Calories: 38 | Fat: 0.1g | Protein: 1.5g | Sodium: 79mg | Fiber: 3g | Carbohydrates: 8g | Sugar: 5g

Beet Colors

Beets come in many colors, from deep red to orange. They also can be white. The Chioggia beet is called a candy cane beet because it has red and white rings. Small or medium beets are tenderer than larger ones. Roasted beets can be enjoyed on their own or flavored with olive oil, salt, and pepper for a simple side dish.

CHAPTER 16

Condiments, Sauces, and Dressings

Avocado Vinaigrette

This basic, mildly flavored vinaigrette dressing is rich in anti-inflammatory fatty acids and vitamin E and is best served with cold dishes.

PREP TIME: 5 MINUTES
COOK TIME: N/A

INGREDIENTS | SERVES 4

½ cup avocado oil

2 tablespoons lemon juice

1 tablespoon raw honey

¼ teaspoon fine sea salt

1 medium ripe avocado, pitted, peeled, and sliced

In a food processor or blender, purée all ingredients together until well mixed. Serve immediately to preserve the bright green color.

Per Serving Calories: 316 | Fat: 31g | Protein: 1g | Sodium: 142mg | Fiber: 2g | Carbohydrates: 8g | Sugar: 4.5g

Brown Avocado?

Even though avocados turn brown when exposed to air for too long, a brown avocado isn't a bad avocado. While it's most appetizing to eat them when they're nice and green, nothing in the nutrients changes as the avocado browns, thanks to the oxidizing exposure to air. It's the same reason why apples turn brown after they've been sliced.

Honey Lime Dressing

This sweet and tangy salad dressing can be whipped together in just a few minutes.

PREP TIME: 5 MINUTES
COOK TIME: N/A

INGREDIENTS | SERVES 4

⅓ cup coconut oil, melted

2 tablespoons raw honey

2 large limes, juiced

¼ teaspoon sea salt

In a large glass jar or small mixing bowl, whisk together all ingredients by hand or pulse with an immersion blender. Serve warm or at room temperature. If refrigerating, allow to stand at room temperature or warm briefly and stir before serving to remix the coconut oil with the rest of the ingredients.

Per Serving Calories: 192 | Fat: 17g | Protein: 0.1g | Sodium: 145mg | Fiber: 0.1g | Carbohydrates: 10g | Sugar: 9g

Raw Honey Power

Raw honey hasn't been pasteurized, which means that it retains more antioxidants and phytonutrients than its processed counterparts. Raw honey is also antibacterial and antifungal, which is why it's often a go-to remedy for sore throats, colds, and other similar ailments.

Paleo Barbecue Sauce

This sweet and spicy barbecue sauce is perfect for making pulled beef or pork, or for marinating any meats before grilling or baking. Make the sauce a day ahead to make the most of the finger-licking flavor.

PREP TIME: 0 MINUTES
COOK TIME: 1–2 HOURS

INGREDIENTS | MAKES 4 CUPS

2 cups Sir Kensington's Ketchup

1 tablespoon Sir Kensington's Yellow Mustard

1 cup water

¼ cup apple cider vinegar

3 tablespoons coconut sugar

3 tablespoons coconut nectar

2 teaspoons dark molasses

1 large orange, juiced

½ tablespoon ground black pepper

1 teaspoon fine sea salt

½ tablespoon onion powder

3 tablespoons Worcestershire sauce

In a medium saucepan over medium heat, combine all ingredients and whisk together slowly as they warm. Bring to a boil and then simmer uncovered on low heat 1–2 hours, stirring occasionally.

Per Serving (¼ cup) Calories: 64 | Fat: 0g | Protein: 0g | Sodium: 448mg | Fiber: 0g | Carbohydrates: 14g | Sugar: 11g

Fever for the Flavor

Want to spice up this barbecue sauce? Add 1/8 teaspoon cayenne pepper and 2 teaspoons chili powder. Want to make it even sweeter? Add the juice of a second orange and a few teaspoons of raw honey. Or try giving it more depth by doubling the mustard.

Bacon Vinaigrette

This savory dressing pairs nicely with sweet-based salads in the classic marriage of sweet-and-salty flavors that has stood the test of time.

PREP TIME: 10 MINUTES
COOK TIME: 10–12 MINUTES

INGREDIENTS | SERVES 4

8 slices bacon

½ tablespoon garlic powder

3 tablespoons raw honey

Juice from 1 large orange

¼ cup balsamic vinegar

1 tablespoon apple cider vinegar

¼ cup avocado oil

½ teaspoon fine sea salt

¼ teaspoon ground black pepper

1. Preheat oven to 400°F. Line a baking sheet with foil. Lay out bacon on sheet and bake 10–12 minutes or until browned and crispy. Remove from oven. Chop bacon and set aside.

2. Carefully drain bacon drippings from the tray into a medium glass bowl. Whisk bacon drippings with garlic powder, honey, orange juice, vinegars, oil, salt, and pepper. Stir in chopped bacon. Serve warm.

Per Serving   Calories: 304 | Fat: 21g | Protein: 8g | Sodium: 671mg | Fiber: 0.2g | Carbohydrates: 18.5g | Sugar: 16.5g

Paleo Slaw Sauce

Turn any combination of vegetables into your own fresh version of slaw by tossing them in this easy slaw sauce.

PREP TIME: 30 MINUTES
COOK TIME: N/A

INGREDIENTS | SERVES 4

¾ cup Homemade Mayonnaise (see recipe in this chapter)

2 tablespoons date sugar

2 tablespoons lemon juice

2 teaspoons apple cider vinegar

½ teaspoon ground black pepper

¼ teaspoon fine sea salt

¼ teaspoon onion powder

¼ teaspoon garlic powder

In a small bowl, whisk together all ingredients. Chill before serving. Keep in refrigerator up to 2 days.

Per Serving   Calories: 403 | Fat: 40g | Protein: 1g | Sodium: 152mg | Fiber: 0.1g | Carbohydrates: 7g | Sugar: 5g

Berry Salad Dressing

*This fruity dressing is the perfect addition to any salad, and as a bonus,
can be used as a spread for Paleo breads or crackers.*

PREP TIME: 30 MINUTES
COOK TIME: N/A

INGREDIENTS | SERVES 4

⅓ cup blackberries

⅓ cup hulled strawberries

2 tablespoons coconut oil, melted

⅛ teaspoon fine sea salt

1 teaspoon raw honey

In a food processor or blender, combine all ingredients and pulse until thoroughly mixed. If the dressing is too thick, thin with water 1 tablespoon at a time until desired consistency is achieved. Serve chilled and keep in refrigerator up to 2 days.

Per Serving Calories: 73 | Fat: 6.5g | Protein: 0.3g | Sodium: 70mg | Fiber: 1g | Carbohydrates: 3.5g | Sugar: 3g

Onion Vinaigrette

This onion dressing works well as a marinade as well as a salad dressing. Let it sit in the refrigerator for at least 4 hours before serving to allow the oil and onion flavors to blend well.

PREP TIME: 4 HOURS
COOK TIME: N/A

INGREDIENTS | SERVES 4

3 tablespoons extra-virgin olive oil

3 tablespoons white wine vinegar

1 tablespoon lemon juice

2 green onions, finely chopped

¼ teaspoon ground black pepper

¼ teaspoon fine sea salt

¼ teaspoon garlic powder

In a large glass jar or medium mixing bowl, whisk together all ingredients. Chill in refrigerator 4 hours before serving. Store in refrigerator up to 2 days.

Per Serving Calories: 96 | Fat: 10g | Protein: 0.2g | Sodium: 141mg | Fiber: 0.3g | Carbohydrates: 1g | Sugar: 0.3g

Sweet Potato "Guac"

Not a fan of avocado? Don't let that keep you down!
This cross between guacamole and hummus will be a hit on any party platter.

PREP TIME: 1 HOUR
COOK TIME: 12–15 MINUTES

INGREDIENTS | SERVES 4

1 large sweet potato, peeled and quartered

3 cups water

2 cloves garlic, peeled and chopped

2 tablespoons lemon juice

1 tablespoon avocado oil

1 tablespoon extra-virgin olive oil

1 teaspoon ground cumin

1 teaspoon chili powder

½ teaspoon fine sea salt

¼ teaspoon ground black pepper

1. In a small saucepan, boil sweet potato in water until soft, about 12–15 minutes. Remove from heat and drain.

2. In a food processor or blender, purée potato with remaining ingredients until smooth. Add more avocado oil, ½ tablespoon at a time, if the mixture is too thick. Chill and serve within 2 days.

Per Serving Calories: 92 | Fat: 7g | Protein: 1g | Sodium: 321mg | Fiber: 1g | Carbohydrates: 7g | Sugar: 1g

Swap Out the Sweets

Try making this recipe with butternut squash, pumpkin, or even cauliflower to change up the flavors or to make use of the vegetables you have on hand. You can even make it a blend of more than one or a combination of several root vegetables or those that soften easily when they're cooked.

Pineapple Salad Dressing

This creamy dressing will have you dreaming of tropical salads,
but why dream when you can whip this up in less than 5 minutes?

PREP TIME: 35 MINUTES
COOK TIME: N/A

INGREDIENTS | SERVES 4

½ cup Homemade Mayonnaise (see recipe in this chapter)

¼ cup unsweetened pineapple juice

1 tablespoon raw honey

¼ teaspoon sea salt

1 teaspoon coconut aminos

In a large glass jar or medium mixing bowl, blend all ingredients using a whisk or immersion blender. Chill in refrigerator at least 30 minutes before serving. Store in refrigerator up to 2 days.

Per Serving Calories: 276 | Fat: 27g | Protein: 1g | Sodium: 182mg | Fiber: 0g | Carbohydrates: 7g | Sugar: 6g

Mango Salad Dressing

This sweet salad dressing pairs well with dark leafy or bitter greens, like spinach and dandelion greens.
Make it ahead of time and store in the refrigerator up to 2 days.

PREP TIME: 6–12 HOURS
COOK TIME: N/A

INGREDIENTS | SERVES 4

1 small ripe mango, peeled, halved, and pitted

2 tablespoons grapeseed oil

1 tablespoon water

¼ teaspoon fine sea salt

2 tablespoons lemon juice

1 tablespoon raw honey

In a food processor, combine all ingredients until thoroughly mixed. Chill at least 6 hours or overnight before serving.

Per Serving Calories: 129 | Fat: 7g | Protein: 1g | Sodium: 140mg | Fiber: 1g | Carbohydrates: 17g | Sugar: 16g

Ginger Salad Dressing

This salad dressing has a bite that pairs well with Asian noodles, stir-fries, or bitter leafy greens.
Make it fresh and use immediately for the best results.

PREP TIME: 35 MINUTES
COOK TIME: N/A

INGREDIENTS | SERVES 4

¼ cup avocado oil

1 large lemon, juiced

2 tablespoons freshly grated ginger

¼ teaspoon garlic powder

¼ teaspoon fine sea salt

Combine all ingredients in a large glass jar or medium mixing bowl, whisking together by hand or using an immersion blender to thoroughly mix. Chill in refrigerator 30 minutes and serve.

Per Serving Calories: 126 | Fat: 13g | Protein: 0.1g | Sodium: 140mg | Fiber: 0.1g | Carbohydrates: 1.5g | Sugar: 0.3g

Spotlight on Ginger

Ginger is highly effective for reducing aches and pains that are associated with inflammatory conditions such as Hashimoto's. As an additional bonus, it can lower cholesterol, balance blood sugar, and even fend off cancer.

Nutty Vinaigrette

This nutty dressing is perfect for savory salads that contain nuts, seeds, and berries,
as well as for marinating poultry or vegetables before roasting.

PREP TIME: 5 MINUTES
COOK TIME: N/A

INGREDIENTS | SERVES 4

¼ cup lemon juice

¼ cup walnut oil

1 teaspoon raw honey

¼ teaspoon fine sea salt

1 tablespoon apple cider vinegar

In a large mason jar or medium mixing bowl, combine all ingredients and whisk thoroughly. Alternatively, use an immersion blender to combine. Store in an airtight container in refrigerator with a lid up to 2 days.

Per Serving Calories: 130 | Fat: 13g | Protein: 0.1g | Sodium: 140mg | Fiber: 0.1g | Carbohydrates: 2.5g | Sugar: 2g

Lemon-Dill Dressing

This traditional dressing is best with fish dishes.

PREP TIME: 5 MINUTES
COOK TIME: N/A

INGREDIENTS | SERVES 2

Juice of 1 large lemon
1 teaspoon fresh dill
½ teaspoon ground black pepper
2 tablespoons extra-virgin olive oil

Place all ingredients except oil in a blender. With the blender running on a medium setting, slowly add the oil. Blend until very smooth. Serve immediately or cover and store in refrigerator up to 7 days.

Per Serving Calories: 125 | Fat: 13g | Protein: 0.1g | Sodium: 2mg | Fiber: 0.2g | Carbohydrates: 2g | Sugar: 1g

Oils

Many salad dressing recipes call for extra-virgin olive oil, but you should feel free to experiment with various Paleo-friendly oils. Each oil has a different flavor and, more importantly, a different fat profile. Flaxseed oil is higher in omega-3 fatty acid than others. Walnut oil has a lower omega-6 to omega-3 ratio compared with others. Udo's Oil is a nice blend of oils with various omega-3s, 6s, and 9s. These oils together have a nice flavor and have the best to offer in a fat profile.

Asian Dressing

Asian dressing is perfect with poultry. When you crave the taste of Chinese food,
add this dressing to any plain dish to spice things up a bit.

PREP TIME: 5 MINUTES
COOK TIME: N/A

INGREDIENTS | SERVES 4

2 tablespoons sesame oil

2 tablespoons coconut aminos

½ teaspoon ground black pepper

1 teaspoon dried thyme

2 tablespoons extra-virgin olive oil

Place all ingredients except oil in a blender. With the blender running on a medium setting, slowly add the oil. Blend until very smooth. Serve immediately or cover and store in refrigerator up to 7 days.

Per Serving Calories: 128 | Fat: 13g | Protein: 0.1g | Sodium: 169mg | Fiber: 0.2g | Carbohydrates: 2g | Sugar: 0g

Paleo Hummus

This is a great alternative to the traditional legume-based hummus.

PREP TIME: 30 MINUTES
COOK TIME: N/A

INGREDIENTS | SERVES 8

4 medium beets, scrubbed, cooked, and cubed

¼ cup raw tahini paste

¼ cup lemon juice

1 small clove garlic, peeled and pressed

Place all ingredients in a food processor and pulse until smooth. Chill in refrigerator before serving.

Per Serving Calories: 63 | Fat: 4g | Protein: 2g | Sodium: 37mg | Fiber: 1.5g | Carbohydrates: 6g | Sugar: 3g

French Dressing

This is a great dressing on a crisp green salad.
You can also use it as a marinade for beef, chicken, or pork.

PREP TIME: 5 MINUTES
COOK TIME: N/A

INGREDIENTS | SERVES 8

⅓ cup red wine vinegar

½ teaspoon Worcestershire sauce

1 clove garlic, peeled and chopped

2 tablespoons chopped fresh flat-leaf Italian parsley

1 teaspoon dried thyme

1 teaspoon dried rosemary

¼ teaspoon raw honey

⅔ cup extra-virgin olive oil

Place all ingredients except oil in a blender. With the blender running on a medium setting, slowly add oil. Blend until very smooth. Serve immediately or cover and store in refrigerator up to 7 days.

Per Serving Calories: 163 | Fat: 17.5g | Protein: 0.1g | Sodium: 5mg | Fiber: 0.1g | Carbohydrates: 1g | Sugar: 0.2g

Italian Dressing

Try doubling this recipe and storing in a glass jar.
It will keep for several days and is much better than supermarket dressings.

PREP TIME: 5 MINUTES
COOK TIME: N/A

INGREDIENTS | SERVES 8

⅓ cup balsamic vinegar

½ teaspoon dry mustard

1 teaspoon lemon juice

2 cloves garlic, peeled and chopped

1 teaspoon dried oregano or 1 tablespoon fresh oregano leaves

½ teaspoon fine sea salt

½ teaspoon ground black pepper

½ cup extra-virgin olive oil

Place all ingredients except oil in a blender. With the blender running on a medium setting, slowly add oil. Blend until very smooth. Serve immediately or cover and store in refrigerator up to 7 days.

Per Serving (2 tablespoons) Calories: 131 | Fat: 13g | Protein: 0.2g | Sodium: 148mg | Fiber: 0.2g | Carbohydrates: 2g | Sugar: 2g

Homemade Mayonnaise

This Paleo-friendly mayonnaise is great on beef, turkey, or chicken burgers.

PREP TIME: 5 MINUTES
COOK TIME: N/A

INGREDIENTS | SERVES 16

2 large eggs
2 tablespoons lemon juice
1 teaspoon dry mustard
2 cups avocado oil

1. Combine eggs, lemon juice, and dry mustard in a food processor and pulse until blended.

2. Drizzle oil into egg mixture slowly and continue to pulse until completely blended. Store in refrigerator for up to 2 days.

Per Serving   Calories: 250 | Fat: 26.5g | Protein: 1g | Sodium: 8.5mg | Fiber: 0g | Carbohydrates: 0.2g | Sugar: 0.1g

Salsa Verde

Tomatillos, a relative of the tomato, are in peak season in the summer and early autumn.

PREP TIME: 15 MINUTES
COOK TIME: 10 MINUTES

INGREDIENTS | SERVES 6

1½ pounds fresh tomatillos, husked
2 medium jalapeños
½ cup chopped fresh cilantro
1 medium onion, peeled and chopped
Juice of 1 large lime
2 teaspoons fine sea salt

1. Preheat oven to 400°F. Rinse tomatillos in warm water and place on a baking sheet with jalapeños. Roast until slightly charred, about 10 minutes.

2. Place tomatillos, jalapeños, cilantro, onion, lime juice, and salt in a blender. Purée until salsa is well blended.

Per Serving   Calories: 42 | Fat: 1g | Protein: 1g | Sodium: 777mg | Fiber: 2g | Carbohydrates: 8.5g | Sugar: 5g

Slow-Cooked Salsa

This may be the easiest salsa recipe ever, and it tastes so much fresher than jarred salsa. If you prefer a milder salsa, remove the seeds from the jalapeños before preparing recipe.

PREP TIME: 5 MINUTES
COOK TIME: 5 HOURS

INGREDIENTS | SERVES 10

4 cups halved grape tomatoes
1 small onion, peeled and thinly sliced
2 medium jalapeños, diced
⅛ teaspoon fine sea salt

1. Stir together all ingredients into a 2-quart slow cooker. Cover and cook on low heat 5 hours.

2. Stir and lightly smash tomatoes before serving if desired. Store in refrigerator for up to 3 days.

Per Serving Calories: 15 | Fat: 0g | Protein: 1g | Sodium: 33mg | Fiber: 1g | Carbohydrates: 3g | Sugar: 1g

Standard U.S./Metric Measurement Conversions

VOLUME CONVERSIONS

U.S. Volume Measure	Metric Equivalent
⅛ teaspoon	0.5 milliliter
¼ teaspoon	1 milliliter
½ teaspoon	2 milliliters
1 teaspoon	5 milliliters
½ tablespoon	7 milliliters
1 tablespoon (3 teaspoons)	15 milliliters
2 tablespoons (1 fluid ounce)	30 milliliters
¼ cup (4 tablespoons)	60 milliliters
⅓ cup	90 milliliters
½ cup (4 fluid ounces)	125 milliliters
⅔ cup	160 milliliters
¾ cup (6 fluid ounces)	180 milliliters
1 cup (16 tablespoons)	250 milliliters
1 pint (2 cups)	500 milliliters
1 quart (4 cups)	1 liter (about)

WEIGHT CONVERSIONS

U.S. Weight Measure	Metric Equivalent
½ ounce	15 grams
1 ounce	30 grams
2 ounces	60 grams
3 ounces	85 grams
¼ pound (4 ounces)	115 grams
½ pound (8 ounces)	225 grams
¾ pound (12 ounces)	340 grams
1 pound (16 ounces)	454 grams

OVEN TEMPERATURE CONVERSIONS

Degrees Fahrenheit	Degrees Celsius
200 degrees F	95 degrees C
250 degrees F	120 degrees C
275 degrees F	135 degrees C
300 degrees F	150 degrees C
325 degrees F	160 degrees C
350 degrees F	180 degrees C
375 degrees F	190 degrees C
400 degrees F	205 degrees C
425 degrees F	220 degrees C
450 degrees F	230 degrees C

BAKING PAN SIZES

American	Metric
8 x 1½ inch round baking pan	20 x 4 cm cake tin
9 x 1½ inch round baking pan	23 x 3.5 cm cake tin
11 x 7 x 1½ inch baking pan	28 x 18 x 4 cm baking tin
13 x 9 x 2 inch baking pan	30 x 20 x 5 cm baking tin
2 quart rectangular baking dish	30 x 20 x 3 cm baking tin
15 x 10 x 2 inch baking pan	30 x 25 x 2 cm baking tin (Swiss roll tin)
9 inch pie plate	22 x 4 or 23 x 4 cm pie plate
7 or 8 inch springform pan	18 or 20 cm springform or loose bottom cake tin
9 x 5 x 3 inch loaf pan	23 x 13 x 7 cm or 2 lb narrow loaf or pate tin
1½ quart casserole	1.5 liter casserole
2 quart casserole	2 liter casserole

Sources

Adams, Case. *Increased Intestinal Permeability, aka Leaky Gut Syndrome.* (Wilmington, DE: Logical Books, 2012).

American Autoimmune Related Diseases Association. "Hashimoto's Thyroiditis." www.aarda.org/diseaseinfo/hashimotos-thyroiditis. Accessed March 12, 2016.

American Thyroid Association. "Thyroid Hormone Treatment." www.thyroid .org/wp-content/uploads/patients/brochures/HormoneTreatment_brochure.pdf. Accessed March 31, 2016.

Archives of Internal Medicine. "Demographic Differences and Trends of Vitamin D Insufficiency in the US Population, 1988–2004." http://archinte.jamanetwork.com/ article.aspx?articleid=414878. Accessed April 1, 2016.

Balch, James F., Mark Stengler, and Robin Young Balch. *Prescription for Drug Alternatives.* (Hoboken, NJ: John Wiley & Sons, 2008).

Blanchard, Kenneth R. *The Functional Approach to Hypothyroidism.* (Hobart, NY: Hatherleigh Press, 2012).

Bowthorpe, Janie A., ed. *Stop the Thyroid Madness II: How Thyroid Experts Are Challenging Ineffective Treatments and Improving the Lives of Patients.* (Dolores, CO: Laughing Grape Publishing, 2014).

Cohen, Suzy. *Thyroid Healthy: Lose Weight, Look Beautiful, and Live the Life You Imagine.* (Dear Pharmacist, Inc., 2014).

Edelson, Stephen B., and Deborah Mitchell. *What Your Doctor May Not Tell You about Autoimmune Disorders.* (New York: Warner Books, 2003).

EndocrineWeb. "Preventing Hashimoto's Thyroiditis." www.endocrineweb .com/conditions/hashimotos-thyroiditis/preventing-hashimotos-thyroiditis. Accessed March 12, 2016.

Greer, Beth. *Super Natural Home: Improve Your Health, Home, and Planet— One Room at a Time.* (New York: Rodale, 2009).

Hadithi, Muhammed et al. "Coeliac Disease in Dutch Patients with Hashimoto's Thyroiditis and Vice Versa." *World Journal of Gastroenterology* 13, no. 11 (2007): 1715–22.

Karren, Keith J., N. Lee Smith, and Kathryn J. Gordon. *Mind Body Health: The Effects of Attitudes, Emotions, and Relationships.* 5th ed. (Glenview, IL: Pearson Education, 2013).

Lahita, Robert G. *Women and Autoimmune Disease: The Mysterious Ways Your Body Betrays Itself.* (New York: HarperCollins, 2004).

LifeExtension. *Disease Prevention and Treatment.* 5th ed. (LE Publications, 2013).

Mangin, Meg, Rebecca Sinha, and Kelly Fincher. "Inflammation and Vitamin D: The Infection Connection." *Inflammation Research* 63, no. 10 (2014): 803–19.

Mateljan, George. *The World's Healthiest Foods.* 2nd ed. (Seattle: GMF Publishing, 2015).

McLachlan, Sandra M., and Basil Rapoport. "Breaking Tolerance to Thyroid Antigens: Changing Concepts in Thyroid Autoimmunity." *Endocrine Reviews* 35, no. 1 (2014): 59–105.

National Institute of Diabetes and Digestive and Kidney Diseases. "Hashimoto's Disease." www.niddk.nih.gov/health-information/health-topics/endocrine/hashimotos-disease/Pages/fact-sheet.aspx. Accessed March 29, 2016.

Northrup, Christiane. "What Are the Symptoms of Estrogen Dominance?" www.drnorthrup.com/estrogen-dominance. Accessed April 2, 2016.

Pizzorno, Joseph E., and Michael T. Murray. *Textbook of Natural Medicine.* (St. Louis, MO: Churchill Livingstone, 2013).

Pyzik, Aleksandra et al. "Immune Disorders in Hashimoto's Thyroiditis: What Do We Know So Far?" *Journal of Immunology Research* 2015: 979167.

Rakel, David. *Integrative Medicine, Third Edition.* (Philadelphia, PA: Saunders, 2012).

ScienceDaily. "Vitamin D Deficiency Related to Increased Inflammation in Healthy Women." April 14, 2009. www.sciencedaily.com/releases/2009/04/090408140208.htm. Accessed March 31, 2016.

Shomon, Mary J. *Living Well with Hypothyroidism.* (New York: HarperCollins, 2005).

Stengler, Mark, James F. Balch, and Robin Young Balch. *Prescription for Natural Cures, Third Edition.* (New York: Turner, 2016).

Vitamin D Council. "Hashimoto's Thyroiditis: Does D Deficiency Play a Role?" www.vitamindcouncil.org/blog/hashimotos-thyroiditis-does-d-deficiency-play-a-role. Accessed April 1, 2016.

Wentz, Isabella. *Hashimoto's Thyroiditis: Lifestyle Interventions for Finding and Treating the Root Cause.* (Wentz, LLC, 2013).

Zaletel, Katja, and Simona Gaberšček. "Hashimoto's Thyroiditis: From Genes to the Disease." *Current Genomics* 12, no. 8 (2011): 576–88.

Additional Resources

Hashimoto's Resources

Hashimoto's Thyroiditis: Lifestyle Interventions for Finding and Treating the Root Cause (Izabella Wentz, PharmD)

HypothyroidMom.com: A website written by thyroid patients and experts with a holistic voice

Stop the Thyroid Madness: A Patient Revolution Against Decades of Inferior Thyroid Treatment (Janie A. Bowthorpe)

SuzyCohen.com: A website with information written by a natural-minded pharmacist with invaluable knowledge of thyroid wellness

Why Do I Still Have Thyroid Symptoms? When My Lab Tests Are Normal: A Revolutionary Breakthrough in Understanding Hashimoto's Disease and Hypothyroidism (Dr. Datis Kharrazian)

Paleo Resources

The Autoimmune Paleo Cookbook: An Allergen-Free Approach to Managing Chronic Illness (Mickey Trescott)

PaleoOnTheGo.com: A Paleo meal plan delivery service

PaleoPlan.com: A website with custom Paleo meal plans, fitness programs, and guided challenges

The Wahls Protocol: A Radical New Way to Treat All Chronic Autoimmune Conditions Using Paleo Principles (Terry Wahls, MD)

Natural Household Cleaning and Body Care

Araza Natural Beauty: Paleo makeup

FATFACE Skincare: Paleo skincare

Klean Kanteen: Nontoxic water bottles

Super Natural Home: Improve Your Health, Home, and Planet—One Room at a Time (Beth Greer)

Toxin Toxout: Getting Harmful Chemicals Out of Our Bodies and Our World (Bruce Lourie and Rick Smith)

MTHFR and Genetic Testing

23andMe.com: Genetic testing

LiveWello.com: Genetic testing information

MTHFR.net: MTHFR information from Dr. Benjamin Lynch

MTHFRLiving.com: A patient-written MTHFR website

SeekingHealth.com: Methylated vitamins for those with MTHFR

Online Sources for Paleo Shopping

http://grasslandbeef.com: Grassfed meat products and more

http://thrivemarket.com: A membership market that offers Paleo foods at discounted prices

www.onestoppaleoshop.com: A source for hard-to-find Paleo Ingredients

www.texasgrassfedbeef.com: Slanker Grass-Fed Meat delivered to your door

www.vitacost.com: An online health food store

Miscellaneous Resources

http://barre3.com: Restorative exercise on the go, available in studios, online, and via an app

http://cronometer.com: Food and nutrient tracking

www.aubreyorganics.com: Organic hair care and body care products

www.ewg.org: Searchable database for toxicity levels of cosmetic and household products

www.fertilityfriend.com: Fertility and hormone charting for women from the convenience of the Internet or a smartphone

Sample Meal Plans

The Paleo diet offers a wide array of flavors that will appeal to any palate. These two 4-week meal plans will get you started on the path to Paleo meal planning, but you'll get the hang of it much faster than you think. If you have specific allergies to foods like eggs, nuts, or nightshades, try starting with the AIP meal plan and seeing how it works for you. These meal plans are designed to make use of leftovers when possible to help reduce the total amount of time that you'll be spending in the kitchen.

4-Week Paleo Diet Meal Plan

Week 1

	Day One	Day Two	Day Three	Day Four	Day Five	Day Six	Day Seven
Breakfast	Apple Carrot Smoothie (Chapter 15)	Chicken and "Grits" (Chapter 8)	Farm-Style Egg Skillet (Chapter 8)	Paleo Pancakes (Chapter 8)	Ginger Green Smoothie (Chapter 15) with 2 hard-boiled eggs	Maple Bacon and Brussels (Chapter 8) with 2 scrambled eggs	Leftovers
Lunch	Shrimp and Chard Salad (Chapter 12)	Teriyaki-Glazed Salmon (Chapter 11) with Asian Broccoli Slaw (Chapter 12)	Ultra Vegetable Bison Stew (Chapter 6) with Old-Fashioned Paleo Biscuits (Chapter 7)	Spinach Chicken Skillet (Chapter 9)	Ham and Chard Soup (Chapter 6)	Savory Chicken and Sweet Potatoes (Chapter 9)	Leftovers
Dinner	Apple Honey Mustard Chicken Breasts (Chapter 9) with Greens and Garlic (Chapter 13)	Filet Mignon and Red Onion Salad (Chapter 12)	Cinnamon Pork Chops and Pears (Chapter 10) with Jicama "Rice" (Chapter 13)	Paleo Mushu Pork (Chapter 10) with Tallow-Roasted Bok Choy (Chapter 7)	Citrus-Cooked Scallops with Spinach (Chapter 11)	Baked Cod with Olives (Chapter 11) with Wilted Spinach (Chapter 13)	Leftovers

Week 2

	Day One	Day Two	Day Three	Day Four	Day Five	Day Six	Day Seven
Breakfast	Peach and Kiwi Protein Smoothie (Chapter 15)	Sweet Potato Chia Pudding (Chapter 8)	Egg and Zucchini Scramble (Chapter 8)	Chicken Bacon Skillet (Chapter 8)	Cleansing Green Smoothie (Chapter 15) with Coconut Kefir Yogurt (Chapter 6)	Simple Breakfast Bake (Chapter 8)	Leftovers

Lunch	"Buttery" Baked Chicken (Chapter 7) with Olive Oil–Braised Brussels Sprouts with Apples (Chapter 7)	Shrimp Curry with Pineapple Relish (Chapter 11) with Cauliflower "Rice" (Chapter 13)	Hazelnut Chicken (Chapter 9) with Garlic-Sautéed Green Beans and Portobellos (Chapter 13)	Mongolian Beef and Broccoli (Chapter 10) with Jicama "Rice" (Chapter 13)	Oven-Roasted Chicken and Brussels (Chapter 9) with Easy DIY Sauerkraut (Chapter 6)	Slow-Cooked Chicken and Mushrooms (Chapter 9) with Sweet Orange Pickled Beets (Chapter 6)	Leftovers
Dinner	Ginger Baked Salmon (Chapter 7) with Beet Green Salad (Chapter 12)	Herbed Chicken, Mushrooms, and Garlic (Chapter 9) with Buttery Steamed Asparagus (Chapter 13)	Beef and Kelp Noodle Soup (Chapter 6)	Slow-Cooker Fish Stew (Chapter 6) with Old-Fashioned Paleo Biscuits (Chapter 7)	Fried Sardines (Chapter 7) with Kitchen Sink Slaw (Chapter 12)	Lamb Burgers (Chapter 10) with Slow-Cooked Radishes and Roots (Chapter 13)	Leftovers

Week 3

	Day One	Day Two	Day Three	Day Four	Day Five	Day Six	Day Seven
Breakfast	Farm-Style Egg Skillet (Chapter 8)	Roasted Vegetables and Eggs (Chapter 8)	Bacon and Parsnip Frittata (Chapter 8)	Apple Carrot Smoothie (Chapter 15)	Ham and Parsnip Breakfast Hash (Chapter 8)	Spanish Eggs (Chapter 8)	Leftovers
Lunch	Baked Mahi-Mahi (Chapter 11) with Roasted Tomatoes, Peppers, and Green Beans (Chapter 13)	Asian Bison and Noodle Bowl (Chapter 10)	Lemon Garlic Chicken Tenders (Chapter 9) with Super Green Superfood Salad (Chapter 12)	Tangy Asian Pork Salad (Chapter 12) with Cauliflower "Rice" (Chapter 13)	Green Pork Chili (Chapter 6)	Zesty Chicken and Green Beans (Chapter 9)	Leftovers
Dinner	Thai Chicken Stew (Chapter 6)	Spiced Chicken (Chapter 9) with Roasted Kohlrabi (Chapter 13)	Roasted Steak and Vegetables (Chapter 10)	Peppery Sautéed Tuna Steaks (Chapter 11) with Skillet-Cooked Vegetables with Lemon (Chapter 13)	Simple Baked Halibut (Chapter 11) with Chopped Zucchini and Peppers (Chapter 13)	Balsamic Steak Sauté (Chapter 10) with Coconut Fried Sweet Potatoes (Chapter 7)	Leftovers

Week 4

	Day One	Day Two	Day Three	Day Four	Day Five	Day Six	Day Seven
Breakfast	Vegetable Hash with Eggs (Chapter 8)	Ginger Green Smoothie (Chapter 15) with 2 hard-boiled eggs	Chia N'oatmeal (Chapter 8) with coconut milk	Sweet Potato and Egg Skillet (Chapter 8)	Chicken Bacon Skillet (Chapter 8)	Cleansing Green Smoothie (Chapter 15) with 2 hard-boiled eggs	Leftovers
Lunch	Sausage and Potatoes (Chapter 10) with Sautéed Turnip Greens (Chapter 13)	Beef Brisket with Onions and Mushrooms (Chapter 10)	"Buttery" Baked Chicken (Chapter 7) with Spicy Potatoes (Chapter 13)	Mango Duck Breast (Chapter 9) with Roasted Cauliflower (Chapter 13)	Ginger Shredded Pork (Chapter 10) with Candied Carrots (Chapter 13)	Broccoli and Pancetta Stir-Fry (Chapter 10)	Leftovers
Dinner	Hawaiian Stir-Fry (Chapter 10) with Jicama "Rice" (Chapter 13)	Chicken Bok Choy Stir-Fry (Chapter 9)	Roast Beef and Baby Potatoes (Chapter 10) with Sautéed Collard Greens (Chapter 13)	Thai Coconut Scallops (Chapter 11) with Lemon-Roasted Broccoli Raab (Chapter 13)	Paleo Spaghetti Carbonara (Chapter 10) with Wilted Spinach (Chapter 13)	Chicken and Vegetable Garden Soup (Chapter 6) with Old-Fashioned Paleo Biscuits (Chapter 7)	Leftovers

4-Week Autoimmune Paleo Diet Meal Plan

Week 1

	Day One	Day Two	Day Three	Day Four	Day Five	Day Six	Day Seven
Breakfast	Chicken and "Grits" (Chapter 8)	Breakfast Root Medley (Chapter 8)	Chicken Bacon Skillet (Chapter 8)	Leftovers	Sweet Potato Chia Pudding (Chapter 8)	Sausage and Potatoes (Chapter 10)	Leftovers
Lunch	"Buttery" Baked Chicken (Chapter 7) with Wilted Spinach (Chapter 13)	AIP Vegetable Soup (Chapter 6) with Old-Fashioned Paleo Biscuits (Chapter 7)	Herbed Chicken, Mushrooms, and Garlic (Chapter 9) with Jicama "Rice" (Chapter 13)	Leftovers	Ginger Baked Salmon (Chapter 7) with Asian Broccoli Slaw (Chapter 12)	Shrimp and Chard Salad, minus tomatoes and eggs (Chapter 12)	Leftovers
Dinner	Baked Cod with Olives (Chapter 11) with Roasted Cauliflower (Chapter 13)	Thai Coconut Scallops (Chapter 11) with Jicama "Rice" (Chapter 13)	Roast Turkey and Asparagus (Chapter 9)	Leftovers	Slow-Cooked Chicken and Mushrooms (Chapter 9) with Wilted Spinach (Chapter 13)	Chicken Apple Patties (Chapter 9) with Roasted Zucchini Sticks (Chapter 13)	Leftovers

Week 2

	Day One	Day Two	Day Three	Day Four	Day Five	Day Six	Day Seven
Breakfast	Ham and Parsnip Breakfast Hash (Chapter 8)	Leftovers	Super Berry Protein Smoothie, minus honey (Chapter 15)	Sweet and Savory Beet Smoothie (Chapter 15)	Sweet Potato Chia Pudding (Chapter 8)	Leftovers	Oven-Roasted Chicken and Brussels (Chapter 9)
Lunch	Citrus-Cooked Scallops with Spinach (Chapter 11)	Leftovers	Lemon Garlic Chicken Tenders (Chapter 9) with Beet, Apple, and Bacon Slaw (Chapter 12)	Chicken Onion Stir-Fry (Chapter 9) with Cauliflower "Rice" (Chapter 13)	AIP Vegetable Soup (Chapter 6) with Old-Fashioned Paleo Biscuits (Chapter 7)	Leftovers	Chicken and Vegetable Garden Soup (Chapter 6)

Dinner	Chicken Bok Choy Stir-Fry (Chapter 9) with Cauliflower "Rice" (Chapter 13)	Leftovers	Roasted Steak and Vegetables (Chapter 10)	Ham and Chard Soup (Chapter 6) with Old-Fashioned Paleo Biscuits (Chapter 7)	Asian Bison and Noodle Bowl (Chapter 10)	Leftovers	Baked Mahi-Mahi (Chapter 11) with Tallow-Roasted Bok Choy (Chapter 7)

Week 3

	Day One	Day Two	Day Three	Day Four	Day Five	Day Six	Day Seven
Breakfast	Chicken Bacon Skillet (Chapter 8)	Sausage and Potatoes (Chapter 10)	Leftovers	Chicken and "Grits" (Chapter 8)	Super Berry Protein Smoothie, minus honey (Chapter 15)	Sweet and Savory Beet Smoothie (Chapter 15)	Leftovers with Fruit and Spinach Smoothie (Chapter 15)
Lunch	"Buttery" Baked Chicken (Chapter 7) with Sautéed Mushrooms with Garlic (Chapter 7)	Chicken and Beans (Chapter 9)	Leftovers	Shrimp and Chard Salad, minus tomatoes and eggs (Chapter 12)	Chicken Apple Patties (Chapter 9) with Arugula and Fennel Salad with Pomegranate (Chapter 12)	Thai Coconut Scallops (Chapter 11) with Lemon-Roasted Broccoli Raab (Chapter 13)	Slow-Cooked Chicken and Mushrooms (Chapter 9) with Sautéed Collard Greens (Chapter 13)
Dinner	Baked Mahi-Mahi (Chapter 11) with Roasted Kohlrabi (Chapter 13)	Roasted Steak and Vegetables (Chapter 10) with Greens and Garlic (Chapter 13)	Leftovers	Roast Turkey and Asparagus (Chapter 9)	Asian Bison and Noodle Bowl (Chapter 10)	Chicken Onion Stir-Fry (Chapter 9) with Sautéed Turnip Greens (Chapter 13)	Ginger Baked Salmon (Chapter 7) with Roasted Radish Salad (Chapter 12)

Week 4

	Day One	Day Two	Day Three	Day Four	Day Five	Day Six	Day Seven
Breakfast	Sweet Potato Chia Pudding (Chapter 8)	Breakfast Root Medley (Chapter 8)	Sausage and Potatoes (Chapter 10)	Leftovers	Ham and Parsnip Breakfast Hash (Chapter 8)	Super Berry Protein Smoothie, minus honey (Chapter 15)	Leftovers
Lunch	Chicken and Beans (Chapter 9) with Jicama "Rice" (Chapter 13)	Lemon Garlic Chicken Tenders (Chapter 9) with Buttery Steamed Asparagus (Chapter 13)	Citrus-Cooked Scallops with Spinach (Chapter 11)	Leftovers	Shrimp and Chard Salad, minus tomatoes and eggs (Chapter 12)	AIP Vegetable Soup (Chapter 6) with Old-Fashioned Paleo Biscuits (Chapter 7)	Leftovers
Dinner	Roast Turkey and Asparagus (Chapter 9) with Super Green Salad (Chapter 12)	Asian Bison and Noodle Bowl (Chapter 10)	Roasted Steak and Vegetables (Chapter 10)	Leftovers	Chicken Bacon Skillet (Chapter 8)	Oven-Roasted Chicken and Brussels (Chapter 9)	Leftovers

APPENDIX D

Paleo Food Lists

Proteins

Anchovies
Bacon
Bass
Beef
Beef liver
Bison
Chicken
Chicken liver
Clams
Cod
Deer
Duck
Duck eggs
Eggs
Elk
Emu
Goat
Goose
Haddock
Halibut
Ham
Lamb
Mackerel
Ostrich
Oysters
Pheasant
Pork
Quail
Rabbit
Salmon
Sardines
Scallops
Shellfish, all kinds
Shrimp
Snapper
Sole

Tilapia
Trout
Tuna
Turkey
Veal
Venison

Vegetables and Fruit

Apples, all kinds
Apricots
Artichoke
Arugula
Asparagus
Avocado
Bananas
Beet greens
Beets
Bell peppers
Blackberries
Blueberries
Bok choy
Broccoli
Broccoli raab
Broccolini
Brussels sprouts
Cabbage
Cantaloupe
Carrots
Cauliflower
Celery
Chard
Cherries
Coconut
Collard greens
Cranberries
Cucumber
Dandelion greens

Dates
Eggplant
Endive
Figs
Garlic
Grapefruit
Grapes
Green beans
Herbs, all kinds
Honeydew
Kale
Kiwifruit
Kohlrabi
Kumquats
Leeks
Lemons
Lettuces, all kinds
Limes
Mangoes
Mushrooms
Nectarines
Olives
Onions, all kinds
Oranges
Papaya
Parsnips
Passionfruit
Peaches
Pears
Persimmon
Pineapple
Plums
Pomegranate
Radicchio
Radish
Raspberries
Rhubarb

Sea vegetables, all kinds
Snow peas
Spinach
Squash, all kinds
Star fruit
Strawberries
Sugar snap peas
Sweet peas
Sweet peppers
Sweet potatoes
Tangelos
Tangerines
Tomatillos
Tomatoes
Turnips
Watercress
Watermelon
White potatoes
Zucchini

Nuts and Seeds

Brazil nuts
Cashews
Chestnuts
Coconut
Flaxseeds
Hazelnuts
Macadamia nuts
Pecans
Pine nuts
Pistachios
Pumpkin seeds
Sesame seeds
Walnuts

Fats and Oils

Avocado oil
Duck fat
Flaxseed oil
Ghee
Hempseed oil
Lard
Paleo mayonnaise
Tallow
Walnut oil

Sweeteners

Coconut nectar
Coconut sugar
Date sugar
Honey, raw
Maple sugar
Maple syrup, grade B
Molasses
Stevia leaf

The Autoimmune Paleo Diet

The AIP allows all the same Paleo foods, with the exception of the following. These should be avoided if you intend to follow this version of Paleo.

Almonds, and all other nuts
Bell peppers
Cacao
Cayenne pepper

Chili powder
Coconut sugar
Coffee
Date sugar
Eggplant
Eggs
Honey
Molasses
Red pepper flakes
Seeds, all kinds
Stevia
Tomatoes
White potatoes

APPENDIX E

Stocking a Paleo Pantry

While it's best to purchase fresh ingredients such as produce and meats one or two times a week (depending on how often you like to shop, or how fresh you like your ingredients—frozen vegetables also work, too!), it is convenient to have a fully stocked Paleo pantry so that when it comes to baking or making other recipes such as soups, stews, or stir-fries, you have every little ingredient on hand. The following list is for a starter pantry, but the longer you're Paleo, the more customized it will become. Another tip: at the beginning of the month, look over the recipes in your meal plan and take note of things like Paleo flours, spices, and cooking fats that can be purchased ahead of time (sometimes even in bulk to save money). Having them on hand will pare down your shopping time because you will only have to round the outer walls of the market for your fresh meats, vegetables, fruit, and eggs.

Cooking Fats

Avocado oil
Coconut oil
Extra-virgin olive oil
Ghee
Lard
Tallow

Paleo Baking Flours

Almond flour
Cassava flour
Coconut flour
Tapioca starch

Sweeteners

Blackstrap molasses
Coconut nectar
Coconut sugar
Date sugar
Maple syrup, grade B
Raw honey

Herbs, Spices, and Seasonings

Black pepper
Cayenne pepper
Chili powder
Cinnamon
Cumin
Garlic powder
Ginger
Himalayan salt
Minced garlic
Minced onion
Nutmeg
Onion powder
Paprika

Red pepper flakes
Sea salt
Turmeric

Nuts, Seeds, Nut Butters, and Nut Milks

Almonds
Almond butter (unsweetened)
Almond milk (unsweetened)
Cashew butter
Cashews
Chia seeds
Coconut milk, full-fat
Hemp seeds
Macadamia nuts
Pecans
Pumpkin seeds
Sunflower seeds
Walnuts

Miscellaneous Cooking Ingredients

Apple cider vinegar
Applesauce (unsweetened)
Balsamic vinegar
Cacao powder (raw)
Coconut aminos
Pickled ginger
Tomato paste
Worcestershire sauce